Cerebral Herniation Syndromes and Intracranial Hypertension

Cerebral Herniation Syndromes and Intracranial Hypertension

Edited by Matthew Koenig

Rutgers University Press Medicine
New Brunswick, New Jersey, and London

Library of Congress Cataloging-in-Publication Data

Names: Koenig, Matthew, 1975– , editor.
Title: Cerebral herniation syndromes and intracranial hypertension / edited by Matthew Koenig.
Other titles: Updates in neurocritical care.
Description: New Brunswick, New Jersey : Rutgers University Press, [2016] | Series: Updates in neurocritical care | Includes bibliographical references and index.
Identifiers: LCCN 2015042930 | ISBN 9780813579313 (hardcover : alk. paper) | ISBN 9780813579320 (e-book (epub)) | ISBN 9780813579337 (e-book (web pdf))
Subjects: | MESH: Encephalocele—therapy. | Intracranial Hypertension—pathology. | Intraoperative Neurophysiological Monitoring.
Classification: LCC RC386.2 | NLM WL 348 | DDC 616.8/0471—dc23
LC record available at http://lccn.loc.gov/2015042930

A British Cataloging-in-Publication record for this book is available from the British Library.

This publication was supported in part by the Eleanor J. and Jason F. Dreibelbis Fund.

Visit our website: http://rutgerspress.rutgers.edu

Manufactured in the United States of America

CONTENTS

PREFACE

Intracranial pressure (ICP) is such a fundamental aspect of neurocritical care that, I would argue, we forget how little we actually know about it. This ignorance has become more explicit over the last few years as the largest randomized controlled trial to date seemingly debunked a pillar of neurocritical care—the need to measure ICP and maintain it under 20 mmHg in severe traumatic brain injury. Anecdotally, any neurointensivist in practice can relay stories of patients with extreme elevations in ICP who were fully conscious and interactive. Indeed, the first lumbar puncture that I performed as a medical student was on a patient with AIDS-related cryptococcal meningitis who talked me through the procedure even though his opening pressure was undetectably high because the cerebrospinal fluid (CSF) overflowed the top of the manometer. Conversely, any neurointensivist in practice can tell anecdotes of patients who herniated or developed massive hydrocephalus with documented normal (or even abnormally low) ICP. These experiences further reinforce the fact that ICP is not a one-size-fits-all property, and tolerable pressure limits clearly differ in various states of disease and normalcy.

Similarly, the concept of cerebral herniation is—on initial inspection—seemingly simple. Like herniation elsewhere in the body, one portion of the brain shifts into an adjacent cavity, thereby compressing surrounding structures. The severity of herniation, however, depends as much on chronicity as the volume of tissue involved or the degree of displacement. Although cerebral herniation syndromes and ICP are clearly interrelated (otherwise, this book would need a different title), the relationship is inexact. As a practitioner, I must confess to having a relatively black-and-white view of ICP and cerebral herniation. I like to categorize disease states into a) those that cause injury due to a global elevation of ICP (ie, diffuse traumatic brain injury, hydrocephalus, high-grade subarachnoid hemorrhage, anoxic encephalopathy with cytotoxic edema) and b) those that cause injury due to focal mass effect, herniation, and the compression of neighboring structures (intracerebral hemorrhage, subdural and epidural hematomas, large ischemic stroke, focal contusions). In this simplified view, the treatment of these diseases should then be primarily directed toward the global reduction of ICP (osmotic agents, sedation and metabolic suppression, hyperventilation, induced hypothermia, CSF diversion) or the alleviation of mass effect (decompressive craniectomy, evacuation of extra-axial hematomas, resection of contused or infarcted brain tissue). Unfortunately, these disease states are sometimes too complicated and dynamic for such a dichotomized approach.

In this book, neurocritical care experts from a variety of neurology, critical care, surgery, and neurosurgery disciplines unravel the complex issues surrounding ICP and herniation syndromes in a concise, practical, and timely review. In planning this book, I specifically chose midcareer authors with specific expertise in these topics, both in research and in real-world clinical practice. These authors work in high-volume centers that treat complex patients with severe traumatic brain injuries and intracranial hypertension as part of their everyday practice and have amassed considerable firsthand experience with the topics about which they are writing.

Although different authors wrote the individual chapters of this book, the book was prospectively designed to flow from chapter to chapter to provide the reader with a cohesive overview of intracranial hypertension and herniation syndromes. Chapter 1 begins with an efficient and practical review of the anatomy and physiology of ICP and cerebral herniation that specifically highlights the areas of discordance and overlap between these two concepts. This chapter provides the basis for the distinct treatments of elevated ICP and cerebral herniation that comprise the later chapters. Chapter 2 focuses on monitoring ICP and the relationship between ICP waveforms and cerebral perfusion and intracranial compliance. Chapter 3 addresses emerging controversies about when and how to monitor ICP, especially in light of new clinical trial data that casts doubt on the primacy of ICP-based therapies. Chapter 4 describes the major cerebral herniation syndromes, the practical signs and symptoms to monitor for impending herniation, and the expected complications and outcomes of herniation events. Chapter 5 and Chapter 6 describe the distinct and overlapping medical management of intracranial hypertension and cerebral herniation, with a particular focus on rapid, disease-specific interventions. Chapter 7 and Chapter 8 describe the surgical management of intracranial hypertension and cerebral herniation, including intracranial and extracranial surgical interventions. Chapter 8 focuses on a systemic approach to treating intracranial hypertension based on recognizing that the human body is really composed of a single compartment artificially separated by somewhat arbitrary boundaries. Chapter 9 closes the book by looking toward the future of neurocritical care, in which ICP—however important—is simply one variable in a multimodality approach to brain monitoring and goal-directed therapies.

I hope you enjoy reading this book. I'm sure that you will learn as much from this book as I did in the process of editing it.

MATTHEW KOENIG, MD, FNCS
The Queen's Medical Center
Neuroscience Institute

CONTRIBUTING AUTHORS

Suhas S. Bajgur, MPPS, MPH
Neurovascular Global Health
University of Texas Health Science Center

Tiffany R. Chang, MD
Assistant Professor
Departments of Neurology and Neurosurgery
Program Director, Neurocritical Care Fellowship
University of Texas Health Science Center

H. Alex Choi, MD, MS
Assistant Professor
Departments of Neurology and Neurosurgery
University of Texas Health Science Center

Indira DeJesus-Alvelo, MD, ABPN
Neurocritical Care Unit
University of Miami Health System

Julia C. Durrant, MD
Assistant Professor
Department of Neurology
Oregon Health and Science University

Holly E. Hinson, MD
Assistant Professor
Departments of Neurocritical Care, Neurology, and Emergency Care
Oregon Health and Science University

Syed O. Kazmi, MD
Department of Neurology
Baylor College of Medicine
Texas Medical Center

Margaret H. Lauerman, MD
Assistant Professor
Shock Trauma Center
Surgical Critical Care
University of Maryland Medical Center

Christos Lazaridis, MD
Assistant Professor
Department of Neurology
Baylor College of Medicine
Texas Medical Center

Scott A. Marshall, MD
Adjunct Assistant Professor
Department of Neurology
Intermountain Medical Center
University of Utah Health Care

Margy McCullough, MD
Department of Neurology
Yale School of Medicine

Chad M. Miller, MD, FNCS
System Medical Chief, Neurocritical Care and Cerebrovascular Disease
OhioHealth
Emergency Neurological Life Support Cochair
Neurocritical Care Society

Kristine H. O'Phelan, MD, FNCS
Associate Professor of Clinical Neurology
Chief, Neurocritical Care Section
Codirector, Neurosciences Critical Care Unit
University of Miami Health System

Starane A. I. Shepherd, MD
Neurocritical Care
Massachusetts General Hospital

Kevin Sheth, MD, FAHA, FCCM, FNCS, FAAN, FANA
Associate Professor of Neurology and Neurosurgery
Division Chief, Neurocritical Care and Emergency Neurology
Director, Neuroscience Intensive Care Unit
Yale University School of Medicine

Deborah Stein, MD, MPH
Associate Professor of Surgery
Medical Director, Neurotrauma Critical Care
Chief, Section of Trauma Critical Care
R. Adams Cowley Shock Trauma Center
University of Maryland Medical Center

Shelly D. Timmons, MD, PhD, FACS, FAANS
Neurosurgical Associate
Director of Neurotrauma, Geisinger Health System
Program Director, Neurosurgery Residency Program
Associate Director for Neurosciences, Geisinger Medical Center Adult Intensive Care Unit
Clinical Associate Professor of Neurosurgery
Temple University

Adam M. Willis, MD, PhD
Department of Neurology
Brooke Army Medical Center

Cerebral Herniation Syndromes and Intracranial Hypertension

1

The Pathophysiology of Intracranial Hypertension and Cerebral Herniation Syndromes

BASICS OF INTRACRANIAL PRESSURE

Kevin Sheth
Margy McCullough

Much pathology of the brain involves a primary injury, such as trauma, infarction, or hemorrhage, as well as further damage in the days following an injury. During this time, the brain is susceptible to secondary insults that are frequently due to increases in intracranial pressure (ICP).

ICP is the pressure within the confines of the skull, which depends on a number of factors. ICP is normally 7 to 15 mmHg at rest for a healthy supine adult, measured at a level equal to that of the foramen of Monro; standing vertically, it typically falls below atmospheric pressure. It is lower in young children (usually 1–7 mmHg), is usually subatmospheric in newborns, and can be up to 18 mmHg in obese adults (1,2). At a steady state, pressure within the brain parenchyma and the intracranial extra-axial spaces is equal, largely due to free movement of the cerebrospinal fluid (CSF) (1,3). Changes in ICP are generally attributed to volume changes in one or more constituents of the cranium.

Under normal circumstances, ICP is maintained in a homeostatic range via intrinsic autoregulatory mechanisms, with occasional transient elevations associated with physiological events that increase central venous pressure and therefore ICP; these may include sneezing, coughing, and the Valsalva maneuver (4). Hip flexion (which decreases venous return), a change in head or neck position, external noxious stimuli, agitation, pain, and seizures can also increase ICP (3). Elevating the head generally leads to a fall in ICP, as CSF moves from cranial to spinal spaces.

ICP sustained at any pressure greater than 20 mmHg is considered pathologic. Based on population studies, ICP greater than 20 to 25 mmHg for a period of 5 minutes or longer poses a threat to adequate cerebral perfusion in adults, and small observational studies have suggested that keeping ICP lower than 20 to 25 mmHg is associated with better clinical outcomes (4–7). ICP in the range of 20 to 30 mmHg is considered moderately increased, whereas ICP that persistently exceeds 40 mmHg is severe and life threatening (1). An observational study reported that mean ICP peaks in patients with traumatic brain injury (TBI) between 2 and 5 days after the initial event (8).

CRANIAL CONTENTS

The cranial cavity, which the inflexible skull and dura protect, has a fixed volume of approximately 1400 to 1700 mL (3,9). Its major constituents include the brain, CSF, and intracranial blood. On average, the brain accounts for approximately 1200 mL of the volume (80% total cranial volume), and the blood and CSF each account for approximately 150 mL (10% total cranial volume each) (6).

Brain

The brain is composed of parenchymal tissue and water; water comprises slightly less than 80% of the brain, 75% to 80% of which is intracellular fluid and the remainder of which is interstitial (3,6). Brain tissue can be classified as either gray matter, also known as *substantia grisea*, or white matter, also called *substantia alba*. Gray matter contains most of the brain's neuronal cell bodies, along with neuropil (dendrites and unmyelinated or myelinated axons), glial cells (astroglia and oligodendrocytes), and capillaries. The brain uses approximately 20% of the body's oxygen, 95% of which goes to the gray matter; it is thus considered the more "active" of the two components. White matter, in comparison, does not contain neural cell bodies and primarily consists of myelinated axon tracts and glial cells.

Supportive septa, or dural reflections, divide the intracranial cavity and protect the brain from excessive movement. They include the falx cerebri, which divides the brain into two hemispheres, and the tentorium cerebelli, which divides the brain into anterior and posterior fossae. The brain parenchyma is largely incompressible and in the absence of pathology generally remains at a constant volume. It has a very small capacity for deformation in the presence of a mass lesion; any pressures exerting a force past that capacity are likely to cause movement of brain tissue into adjacent dural compartments in a process called *herniation*.

Cerebrospinal Fluid

CSF is the extracellular fluid in the ventricles and subarachnoid space that performs a number of major functions in the human nervous system. First, it provides physical support and buoyancy for the brain—CSF's low specific gravity reduces the effective weight of the brain from 1.4 kg to 47 g, which reduces brain inertia and protects against deformation caused by acceleration or deceleration (10). Second, because CSF volume fluctuates reciprocally with changes in the intracranial blood volume, it helps to maintain a safe ICP. Third, because the brain has no lymphatic system, metabolic by-products are largely removed by the capillary circulation or directly by transfer through the CSF. CSF is also important in acid-base regulation and the control of respiration, and it regulates the chemical environment of the brain.

Resting ICP represents the equilibrium pressure at which CSF production and absorption are in balance (11). The average adult has between 90 and 150 mL of CSF within the subarachnoid and ventricular spaces; this volume is smaller in children (3). CSF is produced at approximately 20 mL/hr or a total of 500 mL/day and is in dynamic equilibrium with its resorption (5,6). Most CSF originates from the choroid plexuses, which are located in the floor of the lateral, third, and fourth ventricles; the meninges also produce a small amount of CSF (9). The production of CSF depends upon cerebral perfusion pressure (CPP, discussed in further detail later in this chapter). When CPP falls below 70 mmHg, CSF production falls as well due to reduced cerebral and choroid plexus blood flow. It moves from the lateral ventricles through the foramen of Monro to the third ventricle, via the aqueduct of Sylvius into the fourth ventricle, and then through the foramina of Magendie and Luschka into the subarachnoid space and basal cisterns (10,12).

A hydrostatic gradient passively reabsorbs CSF into the venous system primarily through the arachnoid villi of the dural sinuses, which act as one-way valves between the subarachnoid space and the superior sagittal sinus; some CSF also leaks out around the spinal nerve roots and through the walls of the capillaries of the central nervous system (CNS) and pia mater (3,12–14). The reabsorption process can be described with the following:

CSF drainage = (CSF pressure-sagittal sinus pressure)/outflow resistance

The outflow of CSF is normally of low resistance, so central venous pressure generally determines ICP in healthy patients (15). CSF pressure is highest in the lateral ventricles and decreases as it moves farther down the system (3,9).

Of note, CSF production decreases and reabsorption increases to a slight degree with rising ICP (9).

Blood

The intracranial circulation of blood is about 1000 L/day and is determined primarily by cerebral blood flow (CBF) and cerebral vascular tone (3). Intracranial blood is separated into an arterial component and a venous component; venous blood needs to continually flow out of the cranial cavity in order to allow for continuous incoming arterial blood (16). CBF depends on a number of factors that can be categorized either as those affecting CPP or those affecting the radius of cerebral blood vessels. The Hagen-Poiseuille law, which describes the laminar flow of a uniformly viscous and incompressible fluid through a cylindrical tube with a constant circular cross section, can help explain the factors determining CBF:

$$CBF = (\Delta P \pi R^4)/(8\eta l)$$

Where ΔP is equal to CPP, R is the radius of the blood vessels, η is the viscosity of the blood, and l is the length of the blood vessels.

The brain is unique in that it produces energy almost entirely via oxidative metabolism—thus, adequate CBF to the brain must be maintained in order to both ensure the sufficient delivery of oxygen and substrates and the removal of the waste products of metabolism (17). CBF ranges from 20 mL/100 g/min in white matter to 70 mL/100 g/min in gray matter (which has higher metabolic needs and thus greater blood flow); in an adult brain weighing approximately 1400 g, this equals 700 mL/min, which is equal to approximately 15% of cardiac output (3). The brain accounts for only 2% of total body weight, so it clearly requires more oxygen than other organs; this oxygen requirement is known as the *cerebral metabolic rate for oxygen*, or $CMRO_2$.

Cerebral perfusion pressure

CPP is often used as a measure of adequate blood flow to the brain and is determined by the pressure gradient between cerebral arteries and veins; it can be defined as CPP = MAP − ICP, where MAP is the mean arterial blood pressure and the ICP under normal circumstances is essentially the same as the venous pressure as it exits the skull. CPP is usually around 80 mmHg. As the ICP rises in situations of intracranial hypertension to a level close to that of the MAP, CBF and perfusion decrease significantly due to a decrease in CPP. In general, if CPP is less than or equal to 60 mmHg, there is impaired blood flow to the brain; when CPP is less than or equal to 50 mmHg, mild cerebral ischemia occurs (3). If CPP is less than or equal to 40 mmHg, CBF drops by 25%; CPP less than or equal to 30 mmHg leads to irreversible cerebral ischemia. Hypotension causing a reduction in CPP can provoke a cycle of cerebral vasodilatation, resulting in an increased cerebral blood volume (CBV) and an elevated ICP (9).

Cerebral blood vessel radius

Four factors generally determine the radius of cerebral vessels—cerebral metabolism, carbon dioxide and oxygen levels, autoregulation, and neurohumoral factors. Artery radius is particularly important because it not only acts as the most significant direct determinant of CBF (as it has an exponential effect on blood flow) but can also lead to an increase in CBV, which in turn may separately affect ICP and therefore CPP (18).

Cerebral metabolism. The brain has a significant level of metabolic activity. It requires a continuous supply of glucose and oxygen to maintain energy-dependent pumps that restore and maintain intracellular and extracellular ion concentration gradients, which allow for polarized cell membranes (19). The primary determinant of regional CBF is the metabolic requirement of the cerebral cortex (18). CBF and cerebral metabolism are directly related; any increase in metabolic demand is generally met with an increase in CBF for increased substrate delivery, and an increase in CBF in turn generally leads to an increased metabolism (3). Pathologic states that result in increased cerebral metabolism, such as fever or seizure, lead to an increase in CBF. A number of vasoactive metabolic mediators, including hydrogen ions, potassium, carbon dioxide, phospholipid metabolites, nitric oxide, and glycolytic intermediates, are thought to control changes in CBF and cerebral metabolism.

Oxygen and carbon dioxide. CBF varies directly with $PaCO_2$ and inversely with PaO_2 (20). PaO_2 does not significantly affect CBF in the normoxemic range—with moderate arterial hypoxia or hyperoxia, the unchanged CBF and the unchanged oxygen uptake means that tissue PaO_2 is not a controlled factor (18). However, once PaO_2 drops below 50 mmHg, CBF increases in order to maintain oxygen delivery (18,20). Hypoxia affects vessel radius in a number of ways: it causes the release of adenosine and prostanoids from cerebral tissue, leading to cerebral vasodilatation, and it causes hyperpolarization and reduced calcium uptake in the vascular smooth muscle, which results in an increased vessel radius.

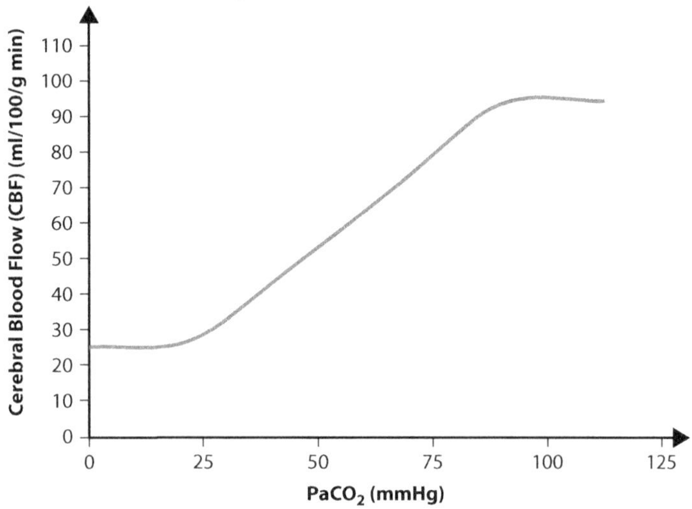

FIGURE 1.1 Relationship between cerebral blood flow (CBF) and $PaCO_2$. The physiologic range of $PaCO_2$ is approximately 20 to 80 mmHg. CBF is most sensitive to CO_2 within these levels and increases almost linearly with an increase in $PaCO_2$.

CBF is much more closely tied to $PaCO_2$ (20), CBF is most sensitive to CO_2 within the physiologic range of $PaCO_2$ (generally between 20–80 mmHg), and CBF increases almost linearly with an increase in $PaCO_2$ (Figure 1.1).

As cellular metabolism increases, CO_2 production increases and causes a dilatation of local blood vessels and increased oxygen delivery; if the cellular activity of the brain decreases, CO_2 production will also decrease and vasoconstriction will occur. Hypercapnia causes intense cerebral vasodilatation, and hypocapnia causes significant vasoconstriction (18). At a $PaCO_2$ of 80 mmHg, the arterioles are maximally dilated, and CBF is approximately doubled. At 20 mmHg, CBF is approximately halved, and arterioles are maximally constricted. Within the range of normal $PaCO_2$, CBF changes by about 4% for each mmHg change in arterial PCO_2.

It should be noted that $PaCO_2$ in the blood also causes an increase of CO_2 in the CSF, leading to acidification of the CSF, which in turn causes cerebral vasodilation, a subsequent increase in CBF, and an elevated ICP (9). Conversely, hyperventilation leading to a decrease in $PaCO_2$ causes an increase in the CSF pH, resulting in vasoconstriction and a decrease in ICP.

Autoregulation. The brain requires a constant CBF over a wide range of pressures. With a CPP within a span of approximately 50 to 150 mmHg, a process called *autoregulation* acts through changes in cerebrovascular resistance (CVR), specifically causing small pial vessels to dilate and constrict to maintain CBF (1,9,19). Emerging evidence indicates that a maximal cerebral autoregulation capacity may be achieved at an optimal CPP of 70 to 90 mmHg (21). Autoregulation is thought to occur by a myogenic mechanism, with vascular smooth muscle constricting in response to an increase in wall tension and relaxing in response to a decrease in wall tension (18). This corresponds to vasoconstriction when the systemic blood pressure is raised and vasodilation when it is low. When blood pressures are extremely high or extremely low, autoregulation fails, and CBF is passively related to systemic blood pressure (Figure 1.2).

The lower limit of autoregulation in normotensives occurs at a MAP of about 60 mmHg—below this limit, CBF decreases, and the arteriovenous oxygen difference increases (18). The upper limit of autoregulation is at a MAP of about 130 mmHg, above which pressures appear to break through the vasoconstrictor response, causing a forced dilatation of arterioles, disruption of the blood-brain barrier (BBB), and edema formation. Of note: autoregulation is generally more effective in maintaining CBF when ICP is elevated than when blood

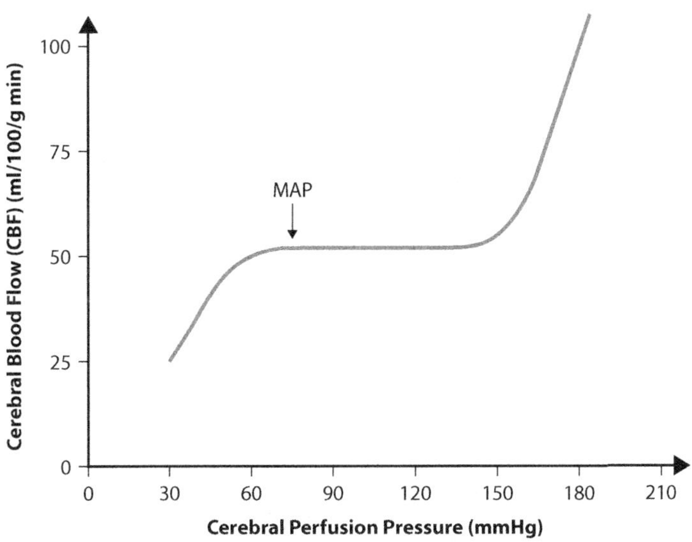

FIGURE 1.2 Relationship between cerebral blood flow (CBF) and cerebral perfusion pressure (CPP). In chronic hypertension, the curve is shifted to the right. CBF is maintained at a relatively constant value when CPP is between 50 and 150 mmHg. When blood pressures are extremely high or low, autoregulation fails, and CBF becomes passively related to systemic blood pressure.

pressure is reduced—low CPP secondary to systemic hypotension is a greater risk than a CPP that results from intracranial hypertension (22,23).

Of further note: the autoregulation curve is shifted to the right in those with chronic hypertension. In these patients, the cerebral vessels have adapted to higher pressure by vessel wall hypertrophy (18). Patients with chronic hypertension tolerate a high arterial pressure better than normotensives. The lower limit of autoregulation of the CBF in patients with chronic hypertension is also shifted to the right, indicating that these patients do not tolerate low MAP as well as normotensive patients.

Neurogenic control. Compared to the body's general circulation, the cerebral circulation has a relative lack of humoral and autonomic control of normal cerebrovascular tone. A network of sympathetic and parasympathetic nerve fibers supplies the arteries on the brain surface and larger arterioles within the brain parenchyma (18). The sympathetic nervous system primarily acts to vasoconstrict and protect the brain by shifting the autoregulation curve to the right in patients with chronic hypertension. The parasympathetic nerves contribute to vasodilatation. However, it has been shown that maximal stimulation of the sympathetic nerves reduces CBF by only 5% to 10% and that a similarly mild vasodilator response to parasympathetic stimulation exists (24–26).

Other factors. As discussed earlier in reference to the Hagen-Poiseuille law, blood viscosity (which is directly related to hematocrit) has a direct effect on CBF—as viscosity decreases, CBF increases. However, the effect of a decrease in viscosity on cerebral oxygen delivery is offset to a degree by a concomitant decrease in arterial oxygen content (27–29). Temperature also has an effect; $CMRO_2$ decreases by 7% for every 1°C fall in body temperature and is paralleled by a similar reduction in CBF, while CBF increases linearly as temperature rises to 42°C (3). Various drugs can manipulate cerebral metabolism and therefore CBF, CBV, and ICP, as discussed in other chapters of this book.

It should be noted that stimuli that cause vasodilatation in a normal brain and lead to an increase in CBF may, in pathologic states, cause a paradoxical decrease in CBF in a so-called steal effect (18). This can happen either globally or locally. Similarly, a stimulus leading to cerebral vasoconstriction and decreased CBF in a normal brain may paradoxically increase CBF in a diseased brain in an inverse steal effect. One example of such a paradoxical stimulus is halothane, a potent cerebral vasodilator that increases CBF in the normal brain and may paradoxically decrease CBF and cause critical ischemia in the diseased brain because of its effect on ICP.

Blood-Brain Barrier

Although not a component of the brain that contributes to total intracranial volume, the BBB is an important structure involved in maintaining total brain volume. The BBB is comprised of intercellular tight junctions between the endothelial cells that line the blood vessels of the nervous system (30). The tight junctions allow only the diffusion of lipid-soluble substances into or out of the CNS and exclude all polar substances. A modified version of Starling's principle applies to the brain as a result of the BBB—in short, excess water and solute are kept out of the parenchyma because water only enters the brain under hydrostatic pressure and without any solute. Because the blood is forced to retain ions and plasma proteins, an opposing force drives water back into the blood.

PRESSURE-VOLUME RELATIONSHIPS AND COMPLIANCE

Monro-Kellie Hypothesis

The Monro-Kellie hypothesis describes the relationship between intracranial volumes and pressures (31–33). After the fontanelles and the sutures close, the brain is enclosed in a rigid container limited by bone, and ICP is distributed evenly throughout the cavity (4,16). The cranium and its contents create a stable volume, so any increase in volume of one of the cranial constituents must be compensated for by a decrease or displacement in the volume of another to maintain a constant ICP (31,32). The CSF acts as an initial buffer to increased intracranial volume, with egress into the spinal subarachnoid space and increased absorption, thus decreasing intracranial volume. Venous blood also compensates to a smaller extent, with venous bed compression and extracranial drainage, in response to intracranial hypertension, leading to decreased intracranial blood volume (20,33). These two compensatory mechanisms are able to maintain a normal ICP for an increase in volume up to 100 to 150 mL; anything larger generally leads to a large increase in ICP (5,34). Conversely, in intracranial hypotension, it should be noted that an enlargement of intracranial venous and arterial structures compensates for a decrease in CSF volume (1).

Pressure-Volume Relationships and Intracranial Compliance

ICP reflects the ability of the intracranial contents to accommodate variations in intracranial volume (16,35). The relationship of volume to pressure is described in terms of compliance or elastance (12). *Compliance* is defined as the change in volume over the change in pressure of a distensible chamber, or the amount of distensibility or "give" that the chamber has for expansion (36):

$$\text{Compliance} = \Delta\text{volume}/\Delta\text{pressure}$$

The term *elastance* refers to the inverse of compliance, or the resistance a chamber gives to the expansion of its volume:

$$\text{Elastance} = \Delta\text{pressure}/\Delta\text{volume}$$

It then follows that if compliance is low (as it is in the minimally elastic intracranial space after compensatory mechanisms have been exhausted), a change in volume would result in a large change in pressure ($\Delta P = \Delta V/\text{compliance}$).

The intracranial pressure-volume relationship can be described by a compliance curve (Figure 1.3) (20). Table 1.1 also outlines the various stages of increasing ICP.

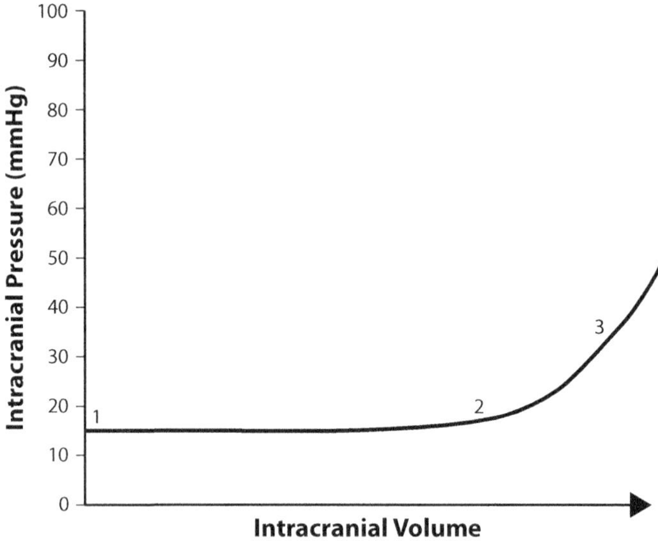

FIGURE 1.3 Idealized intracranial pressure-volume relationships. Point *1–2:* Initial inherent compensation to volume increase with little change in intracranial pressure (ICP). Point *2–3:* Compensatory mechanisms are exhausted, compliance is reduced, and increasing volume leads to increasing ICP. Point *3–4:* Critical volume is reached; small increases in intracranial volume lead to a large increase in ICP at a rate approximating an exponential function. *Note:* MAP, mean arterial pressure.

TABLE 1.1 The clinical stages of intracranial hypertension

	Intracranial Response	Clinical Signs and Symptoms
Stage 1	Increase in intracranial volume met with compensatory reduction in CSF and blood volume—no rise in ICP	None
Stage 2	Exhaustion of compensatory mechanisms, slow rise in ICP	Drowsiness, headache
Stage 3	Rapid rise in ICP with concomitant fall in CPP	Deteriorating level of consciousness, intermittent hypertension, and bradycardia
Stage 4	Cerebral vasomotor paralysis; ICP = MAP, CPP = 0	Coma, fixed dilated pupils, death

Note: CSF, cerebrospinal fluid; CPP, cerebral perfusion pressure; ICP, intracranial pressure; MAP, mean arterial pressure.

The first portion of the graph in Figure 1 (point *1* to point *2*) represents the initial spatial compensation, during which a small increase in intracranial volume causes little to no change in ICP as small reductions in CSF and blood volume act as buffers (12,16,20). In the second portion of the graph (point *2* to point *3*), the natural compensatory mechanisms have been exhausted, leading to reduced compliance. Here, increasing volume leads to a progressive elevation of ICP; this generally occurs around ICP values greater than 25 mmHg. The third part of the graph (point *3* to point *4*) indicates when a critical volume within the cranium has been reached, ICP is already elevated, and small increases in intracranial volume will result in marked increases of ICP; on the vertical portion of the curve, compliance is low and elastance is high (12). Ultimately, as intracranial volume increases, ICP increases at a rate approximating an exponential function.

The rate of change in intracranial volume also affects the ICP: changes in volume that occur slowly generally produce a lesser effect, since the brain has more time to accommodate them, than do rapidly changing volumes (4,12).

Age and Intracranial Compliance

Infants, whose fontanelles and sutures have not yet closed, are known to have significantly increased compliance, as the intracranial space is more distensible during this time of life. Once these structures close, the pressure-volume relationship in children is essentially the same as that seen in adults.

Little official research regarding changes in compliance of the elderly brain has been conducted. It logically follows that compliance is likely to be increased in patients with brain atrophy, thus, theoretically, resulting in greater intracranial space to accommodate increases in the volume of any constituent (15). However, the majority of the published research on compliance in the elderly brain has shown somewhat different findings. Uftring et al showed that aging is associated with a loss of brain tissue compressibility (37), and Albeck et al showed that CSF absorption is reduced in the elderly (38). Czosnyka et al reported a nonlinear *increase* of the elastance coefficient with age in patients with hydrocephalus (39). Kiening et al studied continuous intracranial compliance (cICC) in patients with TBI; they found that the median ICP and cICC did not correlate with the age of individual patients but that cICC was, not surprisingly, significantly reduced with increasing ICP. Patients with the best cICC at high ICPs were in the youngest age group (40). These studies imply that the elderly brain may exhibit an increased "stiffness" and that intracranial compliance may be unchanged or reduced (40). Further research on this topic is needed.

CAUSES OF ELEVATED INTRACRANIAL PRESSURE

It should be noted that many patients with elevated ICP often show concurrent changes in multiple intracranial constituents. Teasdale et al found that in patients with severe diffuse injury and a subsequent increase in ICP, intracranial hypertension was not generally explained by changes in a single intracranial constituent but rather more likely by varying combinations of increased brain water content, CBV, and CSF (41).

Multiple factors govern increased ICP, including the size of a mass lesion (if one exists) and the amount of remaining space in the intracranial cavity. The severity of edema, the patency of CSF pathways, the speed of expansion, and the vasoregulatory mechanisms are also responsible for the degree of intracranial hypertension in a given patient. Table 1.2 details some common etiologies of intracranial hypertension and their general sequelae.

Increases in Brain Volume

An increase in the volume of the brain can occur in a number of pathologies, the most common being space-occupying lesions and cerebral edema.

Space-occupying lesions

Space-occupying lesions within the brain generally fall into one of the following categories: tumors, abscesses, or hemorrhages (9,15,20). The ability of the brain to compensate for an expanding space-occupying lesion depends upon both the rate of expansion and the location of the lesion.

TABLE 1.2 Some etiologies of intracranial hypertension and their sequelae

Condition	Clinical Sequelae
Intracranial tumor	Mass effect, edema
Subarachnoid hemorrhage	Mass effect, edema, disturbed CSF circulation
Intraparenchymal hemorrhage	Mass effect, edema
Abscess	Mass effect, edema
Traumatic brain injury	Mass effect, edema, vasodilatation
Anoxic-ischemic encephalopathy	Edema
Cerebral venous thrombosis	Edema, disturbed CSF circulation
Brain infarction	Edema
Meningitis	Edema
Acute hepatic encephalopathy	Edema, vasodilatation
Acute hypoosmolar syndromes	Edema
Hypertensive encephalopathy	Edema
Reye's syndrome	Vasodilatation

Note: CSF, cerebrospinal fluid.

a. *Tumors:* Intracranial tumors are a common cause of elevated ICP. Because they are slow growing in general, inherent compensatory mechanisms for intracranial hypertension can be maximally utilized as long as the mass does not obstruct the CSF circulation early in the disease (20). It should be noted that many tumors cause secondary edema or hemorrhage, leading to an even further elevation in ICP.

b. *Abscesses:* Patients with abscesses often present with headache, nausea and vomiting, focal neurological deficits, fever, and an altered mental status; many of these symptoms clearly indicate increased ICP (42).

c. *Hematomas:* Acute epidural, subdural, intraparenchymal, or subarachnoid hemorrhages generally expand quickly, leaving little time for CSF translocation as a compensatory mechanism, and are therefore unlikely to prevent early localized or generalized elevations in ICP (20). A resulting decrease in CBV through the compression of vasculature may be an important acute compensatory mechanism in hemorrhage; this vascular compromise could explain the rapid neurologic deterioration seen in patients with intracranial hemorrhage. Increased systemic blood pressure in response to a reduced CPP may lead to the exacerbation of an existing hemorrhage (1). Hoffman et al studied patients with intracranial hematomas and found that posthemorrhage intracranial hypertension is common; they observed that elevated ICP was especially prevalent in younger patients with supratentorial hemorrhage, while patients with infratentorial hemorrhage were less likely to experience intracranial hypertension (43). There was, however, little difference in outcome between the group of patients who had elevated ICP following a hemorrhage and those who did not.

With a more chronic, slowly developing subdural hematoma, the neurologic pattern is more similar to that of the tumor group (20).

Edema

Edema, the abnormal accumulation of intraparenchymal fluid resulting in increased tissue volume, is both a common result and a cause of increased ICP. The increased brain tissue volume that edema causes will inevitably increase ICP. Additionally, edema can be a consequence of elevated ICP—in a compensatory effort to maintain CBF during periods of intracranial hypertension, upstream arterial resistance may be reduced in order to increase CBV. Changes in arterial and venous vascular resistance and pressures may lead to increased capillary pressure and predispose to the formation of cerebral edema (20). It should be noted that conditions that generally lead to peripheral edema (for example, hypoalbuminemia, increased systemic venous pressure) do not cause cerebral edema (9).

Klatzo suggested two major categories of edema with differing pathophysiologies related to physical location: vasogenic and cytotoxic (44,45).

a. *Vasogenic edema* is defined as fluid, originating from blood vessels, that accumulates around cells (46). It occurs when an injury to small blood vessel walls allows the extravasation of intracellular contents, including proteins, into the surrounding extracellular space, particularly that of the white matter (47). The breakdown of these proteins is thought to create an osmotic gradient leading to the movement of water out of the vasculature (44). Its major feature is increased permeability of the BBB with a net gain of fluid in the brain, leading to an increased brain volume and therefore increased ICP (30). More current research also indicates that the active vesicular transport of water across endothelial cells is another important factor (9). Because fluid is able to flow along fiber tracts, swelling in the setting of vasogenic edema is commonly worse in white matter, with its looser structural organization, than in gray matter (9,30). Vasogenic edema is commonly found in patients with brain tumors, meningitis, encephalitis, hypertensive encephalopathy, hepatic encephalopathy, subarachnoid hemorrhage, dural sinus thrombosis, and traumatic lesions (15,20,30). In tumors, tumor cells may produce proteases that act as microvascular transudative factors and cause loosening of the BBB, allowing the passage of blood proteins and contributing to vasogenic edema (9). Small proteins generated by protease action may exert osmotic effects and spread through white matter tracts of the brain, leading to localized edema around a tumor.

b. *Cytotoxic edema* is defined as fluid accumulating within cells due to injury (46). It occurs when the permeability of cellular membranes increases due to cellular injury, leading to the intracellular accumulation of excess fluids and a decrease in extracellular fluid space (9,20). Although swelling occurs in all cellular elements (neurons, glia, and endothelial cells), neurons are most vulnerable to cellular injury, so the effects of cytotoxic edema may be more severe in gray matter than in white. In cytotoxic edema, vascular permeability (and the BBB) is relatively undisturbed, and because water shifts from extracellular to intracellular compartments, there is relatively little mass effect (compared with vasogenic edema) (9,44). Cytotoxic edema generally occurs adjacent to areas of focal or global ischemia and hypoxia, acute hyponatremia, TBI, and Reye's syndrome (15,20,46). In patients with ischemic injury, oxygen deprivation causes failure of adenosine triphosphate (ATP)-dependent sodium pumps within cells, leading to intracellular sodium accumulation and subsequent cell swelling (9). Free radicals form and proteases disrupt cell membranes, leading to irreversible damage (46). Of note: after an infarction, the extent of cytotoxic edema peaks between 2 and 4 days after the initial ischemic event.

Fishman proposed another type of edema, known as *interstitial edema*, which is more of a reference to etiology rather than to physical location (45,46,48).

c. *Interstitial edema* is somewhat similar to vasogenic edema but occurs in the case of a disrupted CSF-brain barrier, typically accompanying obstructive hydrocephalus. Disruption of the CSF-brain barrier leads to the transependymal flow of CSF, which moves into the periventricular tissues in spaces between cells and myelin (9,48). This leads to acute hydrocephalus.

Simard et al have delineated a somewhat different understanding of edema formation specifically in the ischemic brain, identifying another category of edema—ionic edema—and including hemorrhagic conversion as a natural end-stage of a process that initially presents as edema (49). They emphasize the importance of Starling's principle, which states that the formation of edema depends on a driving force, which is determined by the sum of hydrostatic and osmotic pressure gradients, and a permeability factor, which is determined by the ease with which substances can move between the capillary endothelial cells forming the BBB. In describing postischemia edema formation, cytotoxic edema is identified as the process that creates the driving force for the transcapillary formation of ionic and vasogenic edema. It results in the depletion of water and ions from the extracellular space, setting up a new gradient for sodium between the intravascular and the extracellular spaces across the BBB. Cytotoxic edema is a precursor to swelling because, as mentioned before, there is no significant tissue swelling from cytotoxic edema itself. It involves only the movement of osmotically active particles from the extracellular to the intracellular space and no addition of any new constituent from the intravascular space. It is only after the permeability properties of the BBB change that intravascular contents move to the extracellular space and cause swelling. Simard et al describe three phases of ischemia-induced changes in capillary permeability: formation of ionic edema, formation of vasogenic edema, and hemorrhagic conversion. Ionic edema formation—which is the first phase of endothelial dysfunction after an ischemic event—occurs when sodium is transported across the BBB, leading to an osmotic gradient for water and an electrical gradient for chloride. Sodium, chloride, and water all move to the extracellular space to replenish what was depleted during cytotoxic edema formation. This addition of intravascular contents to the extracellular space thus causes tissue swelling. Vasogenic edema occurs next. It is distinct from ionic edema in that it involves a breakdown of the BBB and the movement of plasma proteins into the extracellular space, as described earlier. Simard et al identify the third phase of edema formation in ischemia as hemorrhagic conversion, which occurs after the restoration of circulation and "catastrophic failure of capillary integrity," (49) leading to the extravasation of all blood constituents into the brain parenchyma.

Increases in Cerebrospinal Fluid Volume

In instances of increased ICP, CSF is generally the first-line compensatory mechanism. An initially slow increase in brain volume will lead to the displacement of some CSF within the skull through the foramen magnum into the distensible spinal subarachnoid space; with time, overall CSF content in the cerebrospinal axis is reduced (20). The progressive growth of an intracranial mass or lesion will ultimately lead to the distortion and the blockage of the ventricular system and the subarachnoid pathways through which CSF moves; when this occurs, CSF translocation as a major means of ICP buffering is not possible (20).

Hydrocephalus is the abnormal accumulation of CSF within the ventricular system of the brain; the ventricular system dilates when CSF flow is obstructed (12). CSF can accumulate in circumstances of increased CSF production, decreased CSF absorption, or the obstruction of CSF flow.

1. *Increased CSF production:* The increased production of CSF, the least common cause of hydrocephalus, is generally seen in patients with choroid plexus papilloma. This is a relatively rare diagnosis (20).
2. *Obstruction of CSF flow (noncommunicating hydrocephalus):* Noncommunicating hydrocephalus, which is also known as *obstructive* or *tension hydrocephalus*, occurs with the obstruction of CSF flow within the ventricular system or at the outlet foramina (12,20). It leads to an accumulation of CSF within the ventricles. Common causes of obstructive hydrocephalus include lateral ventricle obstruction by tumors (ie, thalamic or basal ganglia gliomas), third ventricle obstruction (ie, by colloid cyst or glioma of the third ventricle), occlusion of the aqueduct of Sylvius (either due to primary stenosis or tumor), and fourth ventricular obstruction secondary to a posterior fossa tumor (ie, medulloblastoma, ependymoma, or acoustic neuroma) (12).
3. *Decreased CSF absorption (communicating hydrocephalus):* Communicating hydrocephalus occurs when there is impaired CSF reabsorption in the absence of any flow obstruction between the ventricles and the subarachnoid space (50). It is generally thought to be due to the inability of arachnoid granulations in the superior sagittal sinus to allow CSF absorption back into the venous system. The increased ICP is generally evenly distributed with little early brain distortion; neurologic deterioration is slower in these patients compared to those with mass lesions (20). Common causes of communicating hydrocephalus include subarachnoid hemorrhage, bacterial or tuberculous meningitis, or the congenital absence of arachnoid villi (12,20). Infection, hemorrhage, or inflammatory events can lead to scarring and fibrosis of the subarachnoid space.

Increases in Intravascular Blood Volume

Increased intravascular blood flow to the brain, also known as *cerebral hyperemia*, occurs in a number of different situations, including conditions causing cerebral vasodilation, conditions decreasing venous drainage, and hemorrhage.

1. *Conditions increasing cerebral vasodilation:* Increased vasodilation leads to increased CBV. This can occur in hypoxemia—as discussed previously, when PaO_2 is less than 50 mmHg, CBF increases in order to maintain oxygen delivery to the brain (20). It is also seen in hypercapnia—when CO_2 is greater than 45 mmHg, vasodilation occurs and CBF increases. Hypercapnia can occur for a myriad of reasons, which may include the underventilation of a patient during sleep, pulmonary disease, sedation secondary to drugs, shallow respirations, or pressure on the brainstem. Vasodilation also increases in response to many drugs (anesthetics, anti-hypertensives, histamines) (15). Epileptic seizures lead to an increase in regional tissue metabolism, which is met by an increase in CBF (18). The accumulation of lactic acid in the brain, which can occur from even a brief period of inadequate perfusion of brain tissue, leads to a state of cerebral vasomotor paralysis and the abolition of CBF autoregulation. This causes a dilatation of brain arteries and an increase in CBF (51). Lactic acidosis is also often associated with brain edema and BBB damage. It should be noted that the body's response to a fall in CPP leads to an overall increase in the systemic blood pressure and the dilation of cerebral vasculature, which allows for an increase in CBF and therefore CBV. This causes an increased ICP, which will then lead to a further decrease in CPP, a widespread reduction in CBF, ischemia, and infarction.
2. *Conditions decreasing venous drainage:* Although the arterial blood pressure has a somewhat minimal effect due to autoregulation, increased venous pressure does have a significant effect in that it causes an increase of blood volume in the cerebral venous system and therefore a rise in ICP (9). Compression of the jugular veins, heart failure leading to increases in central venous and jugular venous pressures, venous sinus thrombosis, high positive end-expiratory pressure (PEEP), and mediastinal tumors obstructing the superior vena cava are all examples of pathology leading to increased venous pressure which leads to increased ICP.

It is also important to note that normal venous drainage mechanisms may predispose to edema formation and thus elevated ICP—when bridging veins entering the sagittal sinus or extracranial jugular vein outflow tract collapse in order to decrease CBV, this can create a back pressure that is transmitted to the brain's capillary bed, potentially leading to edema formation (20).

Not surprisingly, intrathoracic pressure changes relate to venous return and ICP. Decreased intrathoracic pressure leads to enhanced venous return and subsequent improvement in cardiac output (52). These lead to a decrease in ICP and an improvement in CPP and CBF.

3. *Abnormal focal accumulation of blood in the brain:* This is also known as hemorrhage, which was discussed earlier.

CLINICAL CONSEQUENCES OF INTRACRANIAL HYPERTENSION

It has consistently been shown that elevated ICP after a cerebral insult is associated with a poor outcome (5,53). A number of signs and symptoms classically accompany elevated ICP, some seen in most cases of intracranial hypertension and others in specific syndromes. The major clinical consequences of intracranial hypertension can be broadly differentiated as either mechanical or vascular (54).

General Signs and Symptoms of Elevated Intracranial Pressure

Only headache, vomiting, and papilledema are generalized symptoms specifically secondary to elevated ICP; all others are secondary to tissue shifts due to mass effect (55,56,57).

1. *Headache:* Pressure headaches may worsen with any increase in ICP, such as from coughing, sneezing, or exertion; they are often described as "throbbing" or "bursting." Headaches from elevated ICP are classically worse in the morning, a feature attributed to the rise in ICP during sleep as a consequence of recumbency, mild respiratory depression associated with sleep leading to hypercapnia and vascular dilatation, and also likely decreased CSF absorption (12,56).
2. *Papilledema:* Papilledema is a generally reliable sign of intracranial hypertension but requires several days of elevated pressure to develop (56).
3. *Nausea and vomiting:* Vomiting is classically seen late in the course of increasing ICP and usually occurs after waking, often with the aforementioned morning headache (56).
4. *Visual disturbances and CN palsies:* Numerous visual disturbances and cranial nerve palsies can result from intracranial hypertension, although most are generally seen in the setting of herniation. Pupillary dilatation is generally a sign of the significant progression of increased ICP and is a hallmark of

herniation. Cranial nerve six palsies are common and exist because the sixth cranial nerve is particularly vulnerable to stretching. Cranial nerve three palsies often occur in the setting of herniation of the medial temporal lobe through the temporal notch, leading to stretching of the nerve as it exits the midbrain; it tends to be ipsilateral to the side of the lesion. Cranial nerve four palsy is seen but is generally less localizing. Fundal hemorrhages may develop in response to acute and severe increases in ICP. This is most often seen in patients with subarachnoid hemorrhage or TBI.

5. *Cushing's triad:* A triad of signs that includes increased systolic pressure (including widened pulse pressure), bradycardia, and irregular respirations; it is important to note that Cushing's triad generally presents at a very late stage of intracranial hypertension that indicates significantly elevated ICP and likely herniation (3,56). The downward displacement of the brainstem and the upper cervical cord through the foramen magnum leads to the compression of structures that control cardiac and respiratory function; this is most often in the setting of a supratentorial mass lesion but can be seen in patients with evolving posterior fossa masses.
6. *Isolated hypertension:* The often acute increase in systolic blood pressure following an initial intracranial insult is thought to be caused by a sympathoadrenal response to the initial injury (3). Blood pressure generally trends down to preinjury levels over the course of hours to days and is not, in this situation, connected with the bradycardia or respiratory irregularity seen in Cushing's triad.
7. *Impaired consciousness:* Elevated ICP causes depressed consciousness via global cerebral hypoperfusion and ischemic encephalopathy (58). In the early stages of intracranial hypertension, particularly in the setting of a mass lesion, patients may have subtle fluctuations in consciousness that could reflect deterioration due to local effects of the mass or be secondary to metabolic derangements (3). Ropper et al identified drowsiness as the major clinical symptom in patients actively developing brain edema, followed by asymmetrical pupils (59). Acutely decreased responsiveness is most often due to caudal displacement of the diencephalon and the midbrain (56). It is important in these situations to consider other explanations for changes in responsiveness, including medication effects, fever, systemic infection, or delirium (3). Thus, the entirety of a patient's exam and clinical course should be taken into account when determining whether impaired consciousness in a patient with intracranial hypertension is due solely to increasing ICP or due to one or a combination of other factors. The utility of ICP monitoring will be discussed later in this text.

8. *Autopsy findings:* Pathological findings on autopsy in patients with intracranial hypertension may include tight dura, flattened gyri, compressed sulci, asymmetry of cerebral hemispheres, midline shift, internal herniation (subfalcine/supracallosal, tentorial, tonsillar), external herniation, posterior cerebral artery infarction, posterior inferior cerebellar artery infarction, diffuse hypoxic/ischemic injury, and brainstem hemorrhage/infarction.

Vascular Consequences

Intracranial hypertension itself does not cause brain damage but rather secondarily produces diffuse or focal ischemia (41).

In patients with a hematoma, Galbraith et al showed that ischemia due to increased ICP and brain tissue shift was the major cause of secondary brain damage and clinical deterioration (60). As discussed earlier, any large increase in ICP leads to a critical reduction in the CPP; if uncontrolled, this decrease in perfusion leads to global hypoxia and an overall decrease of cellular activity. Multiple studies have demonstrated the adverse effects of intracranial hypertension and low CPP on mortality and long-term outcome (61,62). As ICP approaches 50 to 60 mmHg, it comes close to the systemic arterial pressure in the circle of Willis vasculature, leading to global brain ischemia and eventually brain death (63).

Ischemia is present at any CPP less than 40 mmHg; some studies have shown that the lower limit of autoregulation in patients with brain injury is actually closer to 70 mmHg (64).

Ischemia has a characteristic course. It initially results in a cytotoxic phase in which energy failure leads to intracellular fluid accumulation in the setting of sodium and potassium shifts between intracellular and extracellular compartments of the brain (46). Persistent ischemia causes the area of impaired metabolism to expand and leads to the irreversible death of the penumbra.

As CPP declines, CO_2 accumulates, leading to vasodilation and a subsequent increase in blood volume, further worsening the elevated ICP. An insufficient oxygen supply and the resulting ischemia will induce further cytotoxic edema and cause even worse elevations in ICP (54). Cerebral hypoxia is associated with drowsiness, agitation, and reduced cognitive skills and often results in a vegetative state or brain death if left untreated (65). Both the cytotoxic and the vasogenic edema that occur in the setting of ischemia peak between 24 and 72 hours after the ischemic event (46).

The complete interruption of CBF to the entire brain, as seen in cardiac arrest, results in the cessation of all electrophysiological and metabolic functions of the brain (66). In global cerebral ischemia, patients generally are unconscious within seconds, with a rapid depletion in intracranial energy stores—glucose stores are generally depleted within 2 to 4 minutes of global hypoxia, and ATP is usually exhausted within 4 to 5 minutes (67). The decreasing activity of ATP-dependent pumps leads to the movement of sodium, water, and calcium from extracellular to intracellular spaces, leading to cerebral edema. The movement of calcium in particular may lead to the release of intracellular enzymes that trigger initiation of the inflammatory cascade, protein and fat destruction, and cellular injury or death. Reperfusion injury also commonly occurs, as restored blood flow distributes the inflammatory mediators and cytokines, leading to further cell death. Measuring lactate production can also confirm existing ischemia.

Localized ischemia may occur in situations such as strokes, where blood supply to a particular area of the brain is cut off, or during herniation events. Acute regional ischemia may lead to mass effect and herniation that causes a further decrease in CBF (46).

Mechanical Consequences

Because the rigid dural reflections of the falx cerebri and the tentorium cerebelli divide the cranial vault into various compartments, increased brain volume in one area may lead to intraparenchymal pressure gradients between the infratentorial and supratentorial compartments or between the hemispheres; a compartmentalized mass effect with pressure differentials can lead to the distortion and eventual displacement of brain tissue from areas of higher pressure to lower pressure in a herniation event (15,35,56). One of the major causes of mortality, secondary to brain herniation, is a cessation of the respiratory drive.

A variety of "herniation syndromes" usually accompany a mass lesion, leading to increased pressure in a single dural compartment and the subsequent movement of tissue into an adjacent compartment of lower pressure (15,36). The most well-known herniation syndromes include subfalcine/supracallosal, transtentorial, and cerebellar-foramen magnum/tonsillar; less well-known herniation syndromes include upward cerebellar-tentorial, diencephalic-sella turcica, and orbital frontal-middle cranial fossa (9). The specifics of these herniation syndromes, including their localizing signs, will be discussed later in this book.

Discordance Between Pathophysiology and Clinical Manifestations of Intracranial Hypertension

All discussion up to this point in the chapter has focused on the mechanisms of elevated ICP and the expected clinical findings that often follow. However, it should be noted that there are countless instances when intracranial hypertension and clinical syndromes do not accompany one another in the manner one might expect. The examples included here are by no means an exhaustive account of the idiosyncrasies between ICP and clinical presentation that are observed in patients.

1. *Acute vs. chronic elevations in ICP:* Briefly mentioned earlier in this chapter, it would logically follow that an acute cerebral insult leading to the rapid onset of intracranial hypertension (such as an acute intracerebral bleed) is much more likely to elicit dramatic symptoms compared to a chronic, slow-growing increase in the volume of an intracranial component (such as a tumor). Even if the elevations of ICP are the same in the acute vs. chronic setting, it is more likely that patients will display the classic sequelae of intracranial hypertension in an acute setting, when the body is less likely to have multiple compensatory mechanisms at its disposal.
2. *Normal pressure hydrocephalus (NPH):* As discussed earlier, hydrocephalus (or increased CSF volume) often causes increased ICP. However, NPH is a relatively common clinical syndrome seen in aging adult patients that is characterized by ventriculomegaly on imaging and clinical findings of gait difficulty, cognitive disturbance, and urinary incontinence (68,69). These patients by definition have normal CSF pressures and normal ICPs.
3. *Large hemispheric infarcts:* As addressed before, ischemic infarcts in the brain can lead to the formation of edema and elevated ICP. However, multiple studies have indicated that patients with infarcts and postischemic edema do not always have concomitant intracranial hypertension (58,70). Investigations have indicated that clinical and radiological criteria, such as marked midline shift, large volume infarctions, and pupillary abnormalities, are more useful in determining whether or not decompressive craniectomy will benefit a patient than the presence of an elevated ICP reading (71). Poca et al described cases of patients with malignant middle cerebral artery (MCA) infarcts who had ICP values less than 20 mmHg despite significant midline shift, large brain infarctions, and neurological deterioration indicative of uncal herniation (70). Frank et al studied patients with large hemispheric infarcts with edema (LHIE) and found that ICP and CPP in most of these patients were within normal limits, despite neurologic deterioration from LHIE mass effect. There is no evidence that global elevation of ICP is involved in the initial clinical deterioration from LHIE (58). A number of posited explanations exist for normal ICP in patients with large cerebral infarcts. One may involve the decrease in CBF and therefore CBV in ischemia, decreasing the volume of one intracranial component and thus allowing for the increase in another (70). Early compensatory mechanisms, as discussed earlier, could also allow for normal ICP values.

References

1. Yuh EL, Dillon WP. Intracranial hypotension and intracranial hypertension. *Neuroimaging Clin N Am*. 2010;20:597–617.

2. Steiner LA, Andrews PJ. Monitoring the injured brain: ICP and CBF. *Br J Anaesth*. 2006;97:26–38.

3. Ropper AH GD, Diringer MN, Green DM, et al. *Neurological and Neurosurgical Intensive Care*. 4th ed. Philadelphia, PA: Lippincott Williams and Wilkins; 2004.

4. Smith ER, Madsen JR. Cerebral pathophysiology and critical care neurology: basic hemodynamic principles, cerebral perfusion, and intracranial pressure. *Semin Pediatr Neurol*. 2004;11:89–104.

5. Sandsmark DK, Sheth KN. Management of increased intracranial pressure. *Curr Treat Options Neurol*. 2014;16:272.

6. Kalanuria AA, Geocadin RG, Puttgen HA. Brain code and coma recovery: aggressive management of cerebral herniation. *Semin Neurol*. 2013;33:133–141.

7. Brain Trauma Foundation. Guidelines for the management of severe traumatic brain injury. VIII. Intracranial pressure thresholds. *J Neurotrauma*. 2007;24(suppl 1):S55–58.

8. Stocchetti N, Colombo A, Ortolano F, et al. Time course of intracranial hypertension after traumatic brain injury. *J Neurotrauma*. 2007;24:1339–1346.

9. Ropper AH SM. *Adams and Victor's Principles of Neurology*. 9th ed. New York, NY: McGraw-Hill; 2009.

10. Han CY, Backous DD. Basic principles of cerebrospinal fluid metabolism and intracranial pressure homeostasis. *Otolaryngologic Clinics of North America*. 2005;38:569–576.

11. Pickard JD, Czosnyka M. Management of raised intracranial pressure. *J Neurol Neurosurg Psychiatry*. 1993;56:845–858.

12. Kaye AH. *Essential Neurosurgery*. 3rd ed. Malden, MA: Blackwell Publishing, Inc; 2005.

13. Portnoy HD, Branch C, Castro ME. The relationship of intracranial venous pressure to hydrocephalus. *Child's Nerv Syst*. 1994;10:29–35.

14. Park JH, Yoon SH. New concept of cerebrospinal fluid dynamics in cerebral venous sinus thrombosis. *Med Hypotheses*. 2008;70:143–147.

15. Mayer SA, Coplin WM, Raps EC. Cerebral edema, intracranial pressure, and herniation syndromes. *J Stroke Cerebrovasc Dis*. 1999;8:183–191.

16. Andrews PJ, Citerio G. Intracranial pressure. Part one: historical overview and basic concepts. *Intensive Care Med*. 2004;30:1730–1733.

17. Siesjo BK. *Brain Energy Metabolism*. New York, NY: John Wiley and Sons; 1978. *Ann Neurol*. 1979;5:308–314.

18. Lassen NA, Christensen MS. Physiology of cerebral blood flow. *Br J Anaesth*. 1976;48: 719–734.

19. Wolfe TJ, Torbey MT. Management of intracranial pressure. *Curr Neurol Neurosci Rep*. 2009;9:477–485.

20. Shapiro HM. Intracranial hypertension: therapeutic and anesthetic considerations. *Anesthesiology*. 1975;43:445–471.

21. Nakagawa K, Smith WS. Evaluation and management of increased intracranial pressure. *Continuum*. 2011;17:1077–1093.

22. Grubb RL Jr, Raichle ME, Phelps ME, et al. Effects of increased intracranial pressure on cerebral blood volume, blood flow, and oxygen utilization in monkeys. *J Neurosurg*. 1975;43:385–398.

23. Miller JD, Stanek A, Langfitt TW. Concepts of cerebral perfusion pressure and vascular compression during intracranial hypertension. *Prog Brain Res.* 1972;35:411–432.

24. Kobayashi S, Waltz AG, Rhoton AL Jr. Effects of stimulation of cervical sympathetic nerves on cortical blood flow and vascular reactivity. *Neurology.* 1971;21:297–302.

25. Alm A, Bill A. The effect of stimulation of the cervical sympathetic chain on retinal oxygen tension and on uveal, retinal and cerebral blood flow in cats. *Acta Physiol Scand.* 1973;88: 84–94.

26. Salanga VD, Waltz AG. Regional cerebral blood flow during stimulation of seventh cranial nerve. *Stroke.* 1973;4:213–217.

27. Frewen TC, Sumabat WO, Han VK, et al. Effects of hyperventilation, hypothermia, and altered blood viscosity on cerebral blood flow, cross-brain oxygen extraction, and cerebral metabolic rate for oxygen in cats. *Crit Care Med.* 1989;17:912–916.

28. Muizelaar JP, Wei EP, Kontos HA, et al. Mannitol causes compensatory cerebral vasoconstriction and vasodilation in response to blood viscosity changes. *J Neurosurg.* 1983;59: 822–828.

29. Muizelaar JP, Wei EP, Kontos HA, et al. Cerebral blood flow is regulated by changes in blood pressure and in blood viscosity alike. *Stroke.* 1986;17:44–48.

30. Kimelberg HK. Current concepts of brain edema. Review of laboratory investigations. *J Neurosurg.* 1995;83:1051–1059.

31. Monro A. *Observations on the Structure and Functions of the Nervous System.* Edinburgh, Scotland: Creech and Johnson; 1783.

32. Kellie G. An account of the appearance observed in the dissection of two of the individuals presumed to have perished in the storm of the third, and whose bodies were discovered in the vicinity of Leith on the morning of the 24th, November 1821; with some reflections on the pathology of the brain. *Trans Med Chir Soc* (Edinburgh). 1824;1:1821–1832.

33. Mokri B. The Monro-Kellie hypothesis: applications in CSF volume depletion. *Neurology.* 2001;56:1746–1748.

34. Levine JM KM. *Traumatic Brain Injury.* Philadelphia, PA: University of Pennsylvania; 2013.

35. Perez-Barcena J, Llompart-Pou JA, O'Phelan KH. Intracranial pressure monitoring and management of intracranial hypertension. *Crit Care Clin.* 2014;30:735–750.

36. Marmarou A, Shulman K, LaMorgese J. Compartmental analysis of compliance and outflow resistance of the cerebrospinal fluid system. *J Neurosurg.* 1975;43:523–534.

37. Uftring SJ, Chu D, Alperin N, et al. The mechanical state of intracranial tissues in elderly subjects studied by imaging CSF and brain pulsations. *Magn Reson Imaging.* 2000;18:991–996.

38. Albeck MJ, Skak C, Nielsen PR, et al. Age dependency of resistance to cerebrospinal fluid outflow. *J Neurosurg.* 1998;89:275–278.

39. Czosnyka M, Czosnyka ZH, Whitfield PC, et al. Age dependence of cerebrospinal pressure-volume compensation in patients with hydrocephalus. *J Neurosurg.* 2001;94:482–486.

40. Kiening KL, Schoening W, Unterberg AW, et al. Assessment of the relationship between age and continuous intracranial compliance. *Acta Neurochir Suppl.* 2005;95:293–297.

41. Teasdale GM, Mendelow AD, Galbraith S. Causes and Consequences of Raised Intracranial Pressure in Head Injuries. In: Miller JD, Teasdale GM, Rowan JO, Galbraith SL, Mendelow AD, eds. *Intracranial Pressure VI.* Heidelberg: Springer Berlin; 1986:3–8.

42. Alvis MH, Castellar-Leones SM, Elzain MA, et al. Brain abscess: current management. *J Neurosci Rural Pract.* 2013;4:S67–S81.

43. Hoffmann J, Goadsby PJ. Update on intracranial hypertension and hypotension. *Curr Opin Neurol*. 2013;26:240–247.

44. Klatzo I. Presidental address. Neuropathological aspects of brain edema. *J Neuropath Exp Neurol*. 1967;26:1–14.

45. Raslan A, Bhardwaj A. Medical management of cerebral edema. *Neurosurg Focus*. 2007;22:E12.

46. Marmarou A. A review of progress in understanding the pathophysiology and treatment of brain edema. *Neurosurg Focus*. 2007;22:E1.

47. Fenstermacher J. Flow of water and solutes across the blood-brain barrier. In: RG D, ed. *Trauma of the Central Nervous System*. New York, NY: Raven; 1985:123–140.

48. Fishman R. *Cerebrospinal Fluid in Diseases of the Nervous System*. 2nd ed. Philadelphia, PA: Saunders; 1992.

49. Simard JM, Kent TA, Chen M, et al. Brain oedema in focal ischaemia: molecular pathophysiology and theoretical implications. *Lancet Neurol*. 2007;6:258–268.

50. Dandy WE. Experimental Hydrocephalus. *Ann Surg*. 1919;70:129–142.

51. Lassen NA. The luxury-perfusion syndrome and its possible relation to acute metabolic acidosis localised within the brain. *Lancet*. 1966;2:1113–1115.

52. Kiehna EN, Huffmyer JL, Thiele RH, et al. Use of the intrathoracic pressure regulator to lower intracranial pressure in patients with altered intracranial elastance: a pilot study. *J Neurosurg*. 2013;119:756–759.

53. Treggiari MM, Schutz N, Yanez ND, et al. Role of intracranial pressure values and patterns in predicting outcome in traumatic brain injury: a systematic review. *Neurocrit Care*. 2007;6:104–112.

54. Stocchetti N, Maas AIR. Traumatic intracranial hypertension. *N Engl J Med*. 2014;370: 2121–2130.

55. Ropper AH. Management of raised intracranial pressure and hyperosmolar therapy. *Pract Neurol*. 2014;14:152–158.

56. Dunn LT. Raised intracranial pressure. *J Neurol Neurosurg Psychiatry Suppl*. 2002;73(suppl 1):i23–27.

57. Lofgren J, Zwetnow NN. Cranial and spinal components of the cerebrospinal fluid pressure-volume curve. *Acta Neurol Scand*. 1973;49:575–585.

58. Frank JI. Large hemispheric infarction, deterioration, and intracranial pressure. *Neurology*. 1995;45:1286–1290.

59. Ropper AH, Shafran B. Brain edema after stroke: clinical syndrome and intracranial pressure. *Arch Neurol*. 1984;41:26–29.

60. Galbraith S, Teasdale G, Blaiklock C. Computerised tomography of acute traumatic intracranial haematoma: reliability of neurosurgeons' interpretations. *Br Med J*. 1976;2: 1371–1373.

61. Stocchetti N, Zanaboni C, Colombo A, et al. Refractory intracranial hypertension and "second-tier" therapies in traumatic brain injury. *Intensive Care Med*. 2008;34:461–467.

62. Vik A, Nag T, Fredriksli OA, et al. Relationship of "dose" of intracranial hypertension to outcome in severe traumatic brain injury. *J Neurosurg*. 2008;109:678–684.

63. Ropper AH. Hyperosmolar therapy for raised intracranial pressure. *New Engl J Med*. 2012;367:746–752.

64. Artru F. Évaluation du retentissement ischémique de l'hypertension intracrânienne. *Annales francaises d'anesthesie et de reanimation*. 1997;16:410–414.

65. Noble KA. Traumatic brain injury and increased intracranial pressure. *J Perianesth Nurs*. 2010;25:242–250.

66. Andersen BJ, Marmarou A. Post-traumatic selective stimulation of glycolysis. *Brain Res.* 1992;585:184–189.

67. Porth C. *Pathophysiology: Concepts of Altered Health States.* 8th ed. Philadelphia, PA: Lippincott Williams and Wilkins; 2009.

68. Rosseau G. Normal pressure hydrocephalus. *Dis Mon.* 2011;57:615–24.

69. Hakim S, Adams RD. The special clinical problem of symptomatic hydrocephalus with normal cerebrospinal fluid pressure: observations on cerebrospinal fluid hydrodynamics. *J Neurological Sci.* 1965;2:307–327.

70. Poca MA, Benejam B, Sahuquillo J, et al. Monitoring intracranial pressure in patients with malignant middle cerebral artery infarction: is it useful? *J Neurosurg.* 2010;112:648–657.

71. Vahedi K, Hofmeijer J, Juettler E, et al. Early decompressive surgery in malignant infarction of the middle cerebral artery: a pooled analysis of three randomised controlled trials. *Lancet Neurol.* 2007;6:215–222.

2 Intracranial Pressure Monitoring and Waveforms

Syed O. Kazmi
Christos Lazaridis

INDICATIONS FOR INTRACRANIAL PRESSURE MONITORING

Intracranial pressure (ICP) is a dynamic entity that a multitude of factors displacing the brain, cerebrospinal fluid (CSF), or the blood compartments of the intracranial cavity can affect. Any process that has an impact on cerebral blood volume (CBV), disrupts the autoregulation of cerebral blood flow (CBF), and/or impairs normal CSF production and absorption can lead to elevated ICP and theoretically indicate monitoring. In 2007, the Brain Trauma Foundation published guidelines for ICP monitoring in traumatic brain injury (TBI) based on level II and level III evidence. This included monitoring for all salvageable patients with severe TBI and an abnormal CT scan of the head. Severe TBI was defined as a Glasgow Coma Scale (GCS) score of 3 to 8 after cardiorespiratory resuscitation; an abnormal CT was defined as showing evidence of hematomas, contusions, swelling, herniation, or compressed basal cisterns. In addition, ICP monitoring was indicated if the patient satisfied more than one of the following in the setting of a normal CT: an age of over 40, evidence of unilateral or bilateral motor posturing, or a systolic blood pressure of less than 90 mmHg (1). More recently, the Milan consensus conference provided expert recommendations for different clinical settings in TBI as follows (2):

1. *Diffuse brain injury:* Monitoring with a normal initial CT is generally not recommended; if the initial findings worsen on follow-up imaging (eg, contusions develop or basal cisterns become effaced), ICP monitoring should be implemented.
2. *Traumatic brain contusions (TBCs):* Monitoring is recommended for comatose patients with TBCs in whom the interruption of sedation for neurological examination is considered dangerous (radiological signs of intracranial hypertension, severe respiratory failure, ongoing emergency extracranial surgery) or when the clinical exam may be unreliable (eg, severe maxillofacial trauma or spinal cord injury). Monitoring should be considered in comatose patients with large bifrontal TBCs and/or hemorrhagic mass lesions close to the brainstem irrespective of the initial GCS score.
3. *Secondary decompressive craniectomy (DC):* Monitoring is generally recommended in order to assess the effectiveness of DC and guide further therapy.
4. Postevacuation of an acute supratentorial hematoma, ICP monitoring should be considered for salvageable patients with intraoperative brain swelling or the following preoperative features: a GCS motor score less than or equal to 5, pupillary abnormalities, prolonged/severe hypoxia and/or hypotension, compressed or obliterated basal cisterns, midline shift exceeding 5 mm, midline shift exceeding the thickness of an extra-axial clot, additional extra-axial hematomas, parenchymal injuries (such as contusions), or swelling.
5. Patients with associated severe multitrauma (thoracic and/or requiring multiple operative interventions) may require multiple anesthetic procedures and prolonged analgesia and sedation. In those patients, sequential neurological examination is difficult, and ICP monitoring should be considered.

The indications for ICP monitoring in non-TBI patients are broadly extrapolated from TBI experience and literature, with minimal direct evidence and little consensus about the specific need for monitoring in these patients (3). In aneurysmal subarachnoid hemorrhage (aSAH), the additional unique indications include obstructive hydrocephalus (4,5), perioperative monitoring, delayed cerebral ischemia complicated by cerebral edema (6), and as a prerequisite to multimodality monitoring. An external ventricular drain (EVD) is the preferred ICP monitor in aSAH patients since it allows CSF diversion. In intracerebral hemorrhage (ICH), the relevant considerations are a volume greater than 30 mL, obstructive hydrocephalus, and the presence of large-volume intraventricular hemorrhage (IVH) (7–9). Monitoring has also been considered in other conditions, including meningitis/encephalitis, hypoxic ischemic injury, ischemic stroke, and hepatic encephalopathy; CT findings of brain edema are often regarded as a potential indication. Decisions about invasive ICP monitoring also may be based on noninvasive data such as the transcranial Doppler (TCD) pulsatility index (10) and/or optic nerve sheath diameter (11). Table 2.1 summarizes the indications for monitoring ICP in a variety of pathologies.

TABLE 2.1 Indications for ICP monitoring

Diffuse brain injury	- Not required if initial CT is normal
Traumatic brain contusions	- Cannot perform frequently or unreliable clinical exam - Large bifrontal lesions or lesions close to brainstem
Decompressive craniectomy	- To assess effectiveness
Postevacuation of acute supratentorial hematoma	- GCS motor score ≤5 - Pupillary abnormalities - Prolonged/severe hypoxia and/or hypotension - Compressed or obliterated basal cisterns - Midline shift exceeding 5 mm - Midline shift exceeding thickness of an extra-axial clot - Additional extra-axial hematomas - Parenchymal injuries
Associated multitrauma	- Requiring multiple anesthetic procedures and prolonged analgesia and sedation
Aneurysmal subarachnoid hemorrhage	- Obstructive hydrocephalus - Perioperative monitoring - Delayed cerebral ischemia complicated by cerebral edema - Part of multimodality monitoring
Intracerebral hemorrhage	- Volume >30 mL - IVH
Ischemic stroke Meningitis/encephalitis Hypoxic ischemic injury Hepatic encephalopathy	- Imaging findings of cerebral edema or tissue herniation - Suggestion of high ICP based on noninvasive studies (eg, TCD or ONSD)

Note: GCS, Glasgow Coma Scale; ICP, intracranial pressure; IVH, intraventricular hemorrhage; ONSD, optic nerve sheath diameter measurement; TCD, transcranial Doppler.

SPECIFIC TYPES OF INTRACRANIAL PRESSURE MONITORS

In 1951 Guillaume and Janny reported the continuous clinical measurement of ICP with the use of an inductance manometer. By the mid-1970s, monitoring by means of a strain-gauge pressure transducer had become standard neurosurgical practice, influenced by Becker and Miller, who used defined clinical algorithms over a 4-year period with 160 TBI patients. In 1981, Flitter wrote that the technique Lundberg used for continuous monitoring—the ventricular catheter and strain-gauge transducer—"continues to serve as a standard against which other devices can be compared" (12).

A ventricular catheter connected to an external strain gauge is the most accurate and low-cost method of ICP monitoring. This method has proven reliable, permits periodic rezeroing, and allows therapeutic CSF drainage and the injection of intrathecal antibiotics. Traditional ventricular catheter external transducer systems allow intermittent ICP monitoring only when the ventricular drain is closed (13). Commercially available ventricular catheters have a pressure transducer within their lumen; these systems allow simultaneous ICP monitoring and CSF drainage (14). Iatrogenic catheter-related ventriculitis and meningitis are potentially life-threatening complications caused by direct catheter contamination during introduction or by retrograde bacterial colonization of the catheter. Reported infection incidences are in the range of 5% to more than 20%. Using closed drainage systems, sampling aseptic CSF, flushing catheters, and promptly removing unneeded catheters can minimize the risk of infections; CSF sampling may predispose to higher infection rates because of repeated access to the drainage system. The need for sampling should therefore be based on specific clinical criteria rather than being a routine surveillance practice. Continuous antibiotic prophylaxis is associated with a high incidence of antibiotic-resistant CSF infections, and its benefits have yet to be demonstrated (15, 16). On the contrary, the use of comprehensive care bundles (17) or antibiotic or silver-impregnated catheters may further decrease the incidence of catheter-related CSF infections (18–20). After removal, the catheter tip should be sent for culture, as bacterial growth is associated with a high risk of secondary meningitis, and antibiotic sensitivity testing based on microbiological analysis can guide therapy (21).

The potential risks of difficult positioning in the presence of cerebral edema, ventricular compression, and obstruction have led to alternative intracranial sites for ICP monitoring. ICP measurements obtained with intraparenchymal transducers (most popular types: Camino ICP Bolt, Camino Laboratories, San Diego, California, United States; and Codman MicroSensor (CMS), Johnson and Johnson Professional Inc., Raynham, Massachusetts, United States) correlate well with the values obtained with intraventricular catheters. Contemporary intraparenchymal transducers may be classified as solid state, based on silicon chips with pressure-sensitive resistors forming a Wheatstone bridge, or of fiber-optic design (12). Although both systems are very accurate at the time of placement, they have been reported to zero drift over time, which can result in an error after 4 or 5 days (22). This problem has been addressed in the balloon-like Spiegelberg transducer, which may zero itself periodically, although its limited bandwidth may make most of the methods used for the ICP waveform analysis impossible (23).

Most clinicians use these devices for a short period of time, and these potential inaccuracies may not be clinically relevant. Intraparenchymal monitors may reduce the infection rate and the risk of hemorrhage and have overall excellent metrological properties (bandwidth and linearity), as revealed during bench tests (24,25). Despite this information, we reinforce the concept that ICP values should be interpreted carefully and in conjunction with clinical and radiological assessments of patients. When a significant discrepancy exists between the monitored number and the clinical/imaging features, rezeroing or replacing the ICP probe should be considered. The cost of these devices is higher than the conventional ventricular system.

Intraparenchymal microtransducer-tipped ICP monitors are sited in the brain parenchyma through a small burr hole and a skull bolt or a specifically designed cranial "access device," which allows the simultaneous monitoring of ICP, cerebral microdialysis, and brain tissue oxygenation (26). The preferred positioning of such devices is the nondominant frontal white matter in diffuse brain injury or the pericontusional parenchyma in focal brain injury. Intraparenchymal pressure probes placed in the hemisphere contralateral to an intracerebral hematoma may dramatically underestimate ICP even in the case of transtentorial brain herniation (13). This last point highlights an important pathophysiologic limitation; generally, uniformly distributed ICP can only be seen when CSF circulates freely between all its natural pools, equilibrating pressure everywhere. When little or no CSF volume remains due to brain swelling, the assumption of one uniform value of ICP is questionable and probably mistaken. With the most common intraparenchymal probes, measured pressure may be compartmentalized and does not necessarily represent the real ICP—that is, ventricular CSF pressure (25,27). Compartmentalized increases in ICP are associated with brain tissue shifts, leading to depressed consciousness from

TABLE 2.2 Differences between EVDs and parenchymal probes

EVD	Parenchymal Probe
Crosses more brain (tip in the third ventricle)	Less invasive (depth of insertion 1.5–2 cm)
Bedside gold standard for pressure measurement	May give compartmentalized ICP readings
Permits periodic rezeroing—easy recalibration	Zero drift over time
Allows therapeutic CSF drainage	No CSF drainage
Allows injection of intrathecal antibiotics	No injection of antibiotics
Intermittent ICP monitoring (traditional catheters)	Continuous monitoring of ICP
	Combine with microdialysis and brain tissue oxygenation
Catheter-related ventriculitis (5%–20%)	Less risk of infection (1%)
Catheter-related hemorrhage (1%–7% largely asymptomatic)	Less risk of hemorrhage (<1%)
Cost effective	Higher cost

Note: CSF, cerebrospinal fluid; EVD, external ventricular drain; ICP, intracranial pressure.

brainstem distortion, bihemispheric dysfunction through mechanical displacement, and herniation-associated vascular compressions (28). Additionally, regardless of what the "real ICP" may be, we may be monitoring a clinically less relevant compartment (Table 2.2 highlights the differences between EVDs and parenchymal probes).

Subdural and epidural monitors (fluid-coupled, pneumatic, solid state, and fiber-optic) and externally placed anterior fontanelle monitors are less accurate. As Douglas Miller wrote, "It is difficult to know when the subdural catheter is under-reading. For this reason, the method is being used less and less" (12).

THE DIFFERENCES BETWEEN LUMBAR AND INTRACRANIAL PRESSURES

Lumbar CSF pressure is more often measured and monitored in hydrocephalus and benign intracranial hypertension. It is important to emphasize that monitoring over a period of at least half an hour while recording pressure and pulse amplitude should be used as a golden standard. Manometric assessment by measuring the height of the CSF column may be misleading, as

CSF pressure may vary considerably over time. The dynamic nature of CSF pressure makes single measurements obtained from lumbar puncture of limited use in diagnosing these disorders (25). It may miss rises in pressure if performed between pressure waves and, in doing so, give misleading results. Furthermore, it gives no information about CSF compensatory parameters, such as resistance to CSF outflow, the pressure-volume index, or the presence/absence of pathological waveforms such as vasogenic waves. Large vasogenic waves are associated with a low cerebrospinal compensatory reserve and are often seen in normal pressure hydrocephalus. Their presence is also said to be positive in terms of prognosis after shunting, and when present for more than 50% of the monitoring period a shunt is indicated. The pathophysiology of these waves is not clear, but they probably relate to oscillations in CBV (29–32). Ideally, in all cases where CSF circulation disorders are suspected the patient should undergo a period of CSF pressure monitoring and a CSF infusion study (33).

WHETHER TO PLACE AN EXTERNAL VENTRICULAR DRAIN OR AN INTRACRANIAL PRESSURE MONITOR

The choice of whether to place an EVD or an ICP monitor depends largely on the requirement for CSF and/or blood drainage, the presence of significant coagulopathy, the need for multimodality monitoring, personal/institutional preferences, and available expertise. Catheter-related complications, such as infection and hemorrhage, are issues that should be taken into account.

A strong reason to prefer an EVD is for its ability for drain CSF; other advantages include the low cost and the possibility of recalibration. Ventricular drains are more invasive, crossing a greater amount of brain; their positioning requires greater technical skill, and they can be very challenging to place in cases of displaced, compressed, or small ventricles. Ventricular size assessment is also important because CSF drainage from EVDs may fail to reduce ICP if insufficient volume of CSF exists within the ventricles, for example, from mass effect. When the aim of the intervention is ICP control, the effect on ICP should guide the extent of drainage. A reasonable initial drainage rate is 10 to 15 mL/hr (34).

Ventriculostomy is generally associated with a greater risk of infection and hemorrhage (not only related to positioning but also to overdrainage) (35). Intraparenchymal devices are less invasive (with a depth of insertion into the brain of 1.5–2 cm) and easier to place. The main disadvantages include higher cost, drift increases with longer usage times, and the inability to recalibrate. Compared to EVDs, their use does not require rezeroing of the system with changes to the head of the bed (36). Positioning the ICP probe on the side of the larger lesion can potentially facilitate the early detection of intracranial hypertension before neurological deterioration (see the earlier comment in reference to compartmentalization) (37). A monitoring limitation of commonly used EVDs is the inability to simultaneously drain CSF and monitor ICP. Episodes of intracranial hypertension have been described during the continuous drainage of CSF (38,39). The placement of a second parenchymal monitor or the utilization of a "double reading" (fluid-coupled plus fiber-optic) EVD catheter could be useful in detecting ICP events that may require therapy without delay (35).

Reported rates of hemorrhage vary (1%–7% for ventricular catheters; less for parenchymal probes), but rarely, such hemorrhages are symptomatic or require surgical evacuation. Modifications of techniques that might reduce hemorrhage risk (eg, via ultrasound guidance) and the utility of routine postprocedural CT scanning merit further investigation (40–42).

In general, placing an intracerebral catheter is relatively contraindicated in patients with coagulopathy (ie, increased prothrombin time/international normalized ratio [INR], partial thromboplastin time, or a platelet count of < 100,000/mcL). Nevertheless, TBI patients with a mild prolongation of INR up to 1.7 have hemostatically normal levels of coagulation factors, and an INR of 1.6 or less is considered acceptable for placing a ventricular catheter following TBI (43,44). Similarly, the use of fresh frozen plasma or other blood products to normalize clotting parameters before insertion can delay ICP monitoring and is not supported by available evidence (45). In cases of major coagulopathy (eg, due to liver failure or anticoagulant intake), coagulation factor concentrates are often used for rapid correction before placement.

Risk factors for infection include a longer duration of monitoring, the presence of an open skull fracture with leakage of CSF, and leakage around the ventriculostomy site (46). A recent meta-analysis of 23 retrospective studies reported a cumulative rate of positive CSF cultures of 8.8% per patient and 8.1% per EVD (47). It has been claimed that the majority of EVD-related infections occur within the first week after insertion, but recent studies identified a later peak of infection occurring even after 2 weeks, particularly in patients with prolonged EVD placement due to severe intracranial disease (48).

Koskinen et al identified all patients who had their ICP monitored using a CMS device between 2002 and 2010 (49). The medical records and postimplantation

CT scans were analyzed for occurrence of infection, hemorrhage, and insertion depth; 549 patients were monitored using 650 devices. The mean monitoring time was 7.0 plus or minus 4.9 days, with a mean implantation depth of 21.3 plus or minus 11.1 mm (0–88 mm). In 27 of these patients, a hematoma was identified; 26 of these were less than 1 ml, and one was 8 ml. No clinically significant bleeding was found. No statistically significant increase occurred in the number of hemorrhages in presumed coagulopathic patients. The infection rate was 0.6%, and the calculated infection rate per 1,000 catheter days was 0.8. The authors concluded that the risk of hemorrhagic and infectious complications when using the CMS for ICP monitoring is low. The depth of insertion varies considerably and should be taken into account if patients are treated with head elevation, since the pressure is measured at the tip of the sensor. They recommended the use of a parenchymal device rather than an EVD. Where ICP is monitored using parenchymal systems, the use of subsequent ventriculostomy for CSF drainage is suitable as a second-tier therapy. Removal is indicated when ICP has been normal for 48 to 72 hours after the withdrawal of ICP therapy.

The Influence of Transducer Position Along the Phlebostatic Axis on Intracranial Pressure and Cerebral Perfusion Pressure Measurement

In 1959 Lassen defined cerebral perfusion pressure (CPP) based on "arterial blood pressure measured at the level of the head," ie, the midbrain, using the tragus as an external landmark (50). However, mean arterial blood pressure (MAP) is commonly measured at the right atrium (RA). When the head of the bed is elevated 50 degrees, MAP measured at the RA may be higher than that measured at the level of the tragus by up to 18 mmHg, thereby overestimating actual CPP (51). This MAP difference can be even further exaggerated when the head of the bed is more elevated, or the patient is very tall. Failing to appreciate this can produce serious consequences. In neuroanesthesia, it is standard practice during sitting craniotomies to place the blood pressure transducer at the level of the head. Kosty et al reviewed foundational literature and sent an e-mail survey to members of the Neurocritical Care Society (NCS) (52). Of 32 articles reporting CPP data, the reference point for MAP was identified in 16: 10, heart and 6, midbrain. Responses from 31 of 34 United Council for Neurologic Subspecialties fellowship–accredited neurointensive care units indicated the reference point was most often the heart (74%), followed by the midbrain (16%). Conflicting answers were received from 10%. Olson et al also surveyed members of the NCS and found a broad range of opinions regarding the correct reference point for leveling the ICP transducer (53). There were 109 (48.4%) respondents who level to the tragus, 77 (34.2%) who level to the external auditory meatus (EAM), 12 (5.3%) to the tip of the ear, 23 (10.2%) midway between the outer canthus and the tip of the ear, and 4 (1.8%) who level to the outer canthus of the eye. When the sample was restricted to attending physicians (*n*=163), 48.6% level to the tragus, 35.4% to the EAM, 4.9% to the tip of the ear, 10.4% to midway between the ear and the outer canthus, and 0.7% to the outer canthus of the eye.

When knowledge and monitoring of CPP is of the essence, we recommend leveling MAP to the tragus since this is the arterial pressure that "the brain sees." Nevertheless, it is important to recognize that regardless of the actual reference point chosen, it should be consistently applied and that when using the phlebostatic axis as a reference, CPP may be overestimated.

Issues With Zeroing and Leveling Intracranial Pressure Monitors

The practice of monitoring ICP via EVD requires the external strain-gauge transducer to be zero referenced (calibrated) before an ICP value is displayed. Olson et al, in the aforementioned survey of the NCS, also examined the process of zeroing and leveling in the measurement of ICP (53). Most respondents chose either the tragus of the ear or the EAM; although not identical, they are anatomically close and accounted for a combined 82% of all responses.

The Origin of Intracranial Pressure Waveforms

ICP is derived from the circulation of cerebral blood and CSF. The vascular component is thought to derive from the pulsation of CBV detected and averaged by nonlinear mechanisms. More generally, multiple variables such as the arterial pressure, autoregulation, and cerebral venous outflow all contribute to the vascular component (25). The other circulatory CSF component may be expressed using Davson's equation:

$$\begin{aligned} ICP_{CSF} &= (\text{resistance to CSF outflow}) \times (\text{CSF formation}) \\ &\quad + (\text{pressure in sagittal sinus}) \ (54). \end{aligned}$$

The ICP waveform consists of three components, which overlap in the time domain but can be separated in the frequency domain (Figure 2.1).

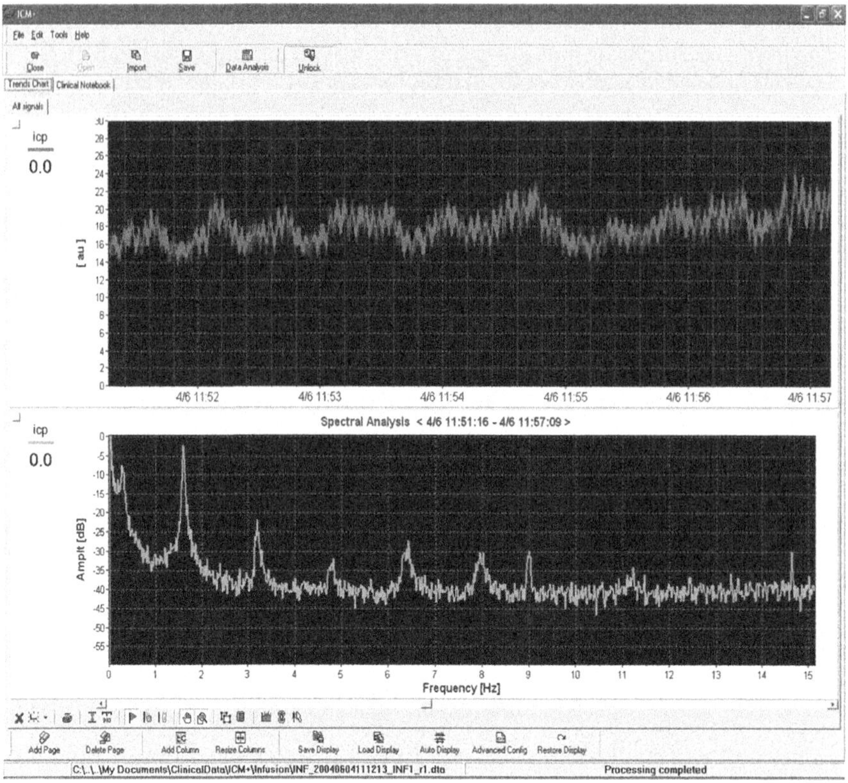

FIGURE 2.1 Spectral analysis and frequency graphs. The upper panel shows the time-domain analysis, and the lower panel shows the frequency-domain analysis of the intracranial pressure (ICP) waveform.

The pulse waveform has several harmonic components; of these, the fundamental component has a frequency equal to the heart rate. The amplitude of this component (AMP) is useful for the evaluation of various indices. The respiratory waveform is related to the frequency of the respiratory cycle (8–20 cycles per minute). "Slow waves" are usually not as precisely defined as in the original Lundberg thesis (55). All components that have a spectral representation within the frequency limits of 0.05 to 0.0055 Hz (20-second to 3-minute period) can be classified as slow waves (25).

Intracranial Pressure Fluctuations and Lundberg Waves

Nils Lundberg's work (1965) on the use of bedside strain-gauge manometers to record ICP continuously by ventriculostomy in more than 400 patients is a

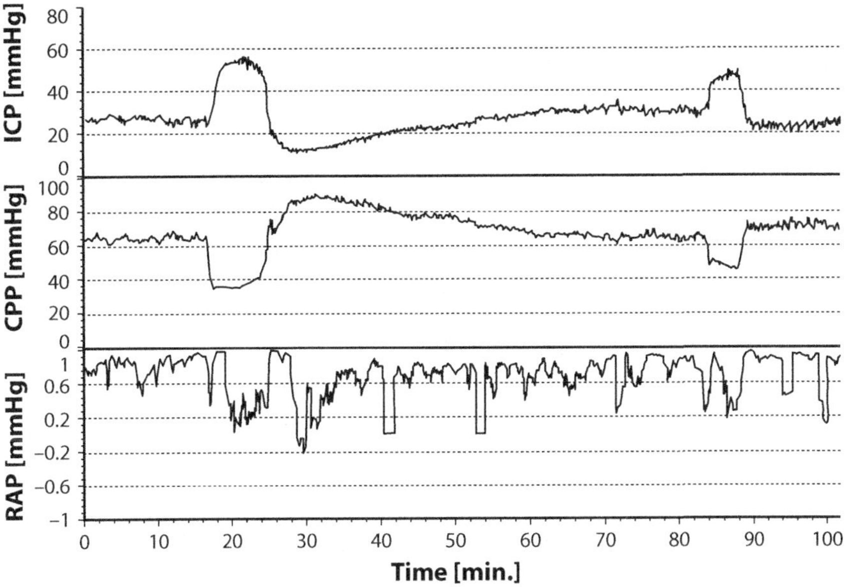

FIGURE 2.2 Intracranial pressure (ICP), central perfusion pressure (CPP), and RAP graphs. ICP plateau waves can be seen with a corresponding CPP decrease.

milestone in the history of ICP recording. Lundberg, anticipating modern practice, wrote in 1965: "The greatest value of recording the ventricular fluid pressure is the information it gives in cases of severe injury of the brain without hematoma. In these cases, intervention to decrease ICP by such means as hypertonic solutions, hyperventilation, hypothermia, drainage of fluid and removal of localized contusions, may be more rationally applied" (12). The waves Lundberg described were (56):

1. A waves, or "plateau waves," have amplitudes of 50 to 100 mmHg lasting 5 to 20 minutes. These waves are always associated with intracranial pathology. During such waves, it is common to observe evidence of early herniation, including bradycardia and hypertension. The etiology is uncertain, but it is postulated that as CPP becomes inadequate to meet metabolic demand, cerebral vasodilatation ensues and CBV increases. This leads to a vicious hemodynamic circle with further CPP decrease (Figure 2.2).
2. B waves have amplitudes up to 50 mmHg with a frequency of 0.5 to 2 per minute and are thought to be due to vasomotor tone instability.

3. C waves are up to 20 mmHg in amplitude and have a frequency of 4 to 8 per minute. These waves have been documented in healthy individuals and are thought to occur because of the interaction between the cardiac and the respiratory cycles. Both A and B waves require intervention to reduce ICP and preserve CPP.

Czosnyka et al continuously monitored ICP to investigate the hemodynamic profile and the clinical consequences of plateau waves in 160 head-injured patients; almost 20% of these patients exhibited plateau waves (57). In 96 patients, arterial pressure, ICP, and TCD blood flow velocity (FV) were studied daily for 20 minutes to 3 hours. Sixteen episodes of plateau waves in eight patients were recorded and analyzed. A profound fall in CPP (by 45%) followed a dramatic increase in ICP; in contrast, FV fell by only 20%. Autoregulation was documented to be intact both before and after the plateau but was disturbed during the wave. The pressure-volume compensatory reserve was always depleted before the wave. Cerebrovascular resistance decreased during the wave by 60%, and TCD pulsatility increased. Plateau waves did not increase the probability of an unfavorable outcome in this cohort. This study is important in showing that plateau waves are a hemodynamic phenomenon associated with cerebrovascular vasodilation; prerequisites for the wave (at onset) are preserved pressure autoregulation and exhausted pressure-volume compensatory reserve.

As mentioned above, the ICP waveform includes three distinct quasi-periodic components: heart rate pulse, respiratory waves, and slow vasogenic waves. Although these components overlap on a background of randomly changing mean ICP, they can be isolated and quantified using spectral analysis. By definition, a frequency spectrum is a graph showing the intensity of individual phasic components plotted against their specific frequency. In the case of the ICP waveform, the area under the curve can be used to quantify the magnitude of each specific component at its characteristic range (ie, heart rate 50–180 beats per minute, respiratory waves 8–20 cycles per minute, and slow waves 0.3–3 cycles per minute). The pulse waveform has a fundamental frequency equivalent to the heart rate and several harmonic components (58). The amplitude of the AMP is potentially more closely linked to intracranial compliance than the mean ICP (pulsatile vs. static ICP) (59,60). Newer indices exploring the association between AMP and MAP (pressure-amplitude index [Pax]) (61) as well as the association between the amplitudes of cardiac beat–induced single ICP and arterial blood pressure (ABP) waves (ICP-ABP amplitude correlation

[IAAC]) (62) may be helpful prognostically and in assessing optimal CPP (CPPopt). Eide et al analyzed cardiac-induced, single wave ICP-ABP pairs to calculate a moving correlation of ICP-ABP wave amplitude correlation (IAAC) as an index of cerebrovascular pressure reactivity in patients with aSAH (62). In patients with an average IAAC of greater than 0.2, mortality was approximately threefold higher than in those with an IAAC of less than 0.2. The same authors had demonstrated earlier, in a randomized controlled trial (RCT), that a strategy targeted in reducing the mean amplitude of pulsatile ICP to less than 5 mmHg vs. a mean static ICP of less than 20 mmHg improved the outcome in patients with aSAH (63). If these findings are reproduced and validated, IAAC may prove to be an important new parameter in optimizing high-grade aSAH patients with compromised intracranial compliance, as well as a parameter to be tested in TBI patients.

PRx, Autoregulation, and Cerebral Vasomotor Reactivity

The operative mechanisms in the regulation of CBF consist of flow-metabolism coupling, chemoregulation (via the acid-base status of the perivascular tissue), autonomic neurogenic control, and cerebrovascular pressure reactivity. Meeting energy/metabolic requirements of brain tissue depends on matching delivery to demand as well as on the functional state of neuronal mitochondria. Mechanisms of flow regulation are paramount in the injured brain's effort to meet these needs and are considered a major innate protective mechanism. A large part of neurocritical care is centered on the manipulation and "optimization" of these mechanisms (64).

Pressure reactivity describes the response of endothelial smooth muscle to transmural pressure. The alteration of vascular diameter, in the arteriolar microcirculation, directly affects arteriolar CBV and, under conditions of a steep pressure-volume curve, ICP. If pressure reactivity is intact, a rise in MAP will lead to vasoconstriction with a reduction in CBV within 5 to 15 seconds, and as a result ICP will decrease. If it is defective, CBV will increase passively and ICP will rise. The opposite applies to a reduction in MAP. These rules do not apply in all instances, for example, when the change in MAP is very fast or large or in conditions of high cerebrospinal compensatory reserve (eg, DC).

The status of pressure autoregulation carries prognostic information in patients with severe TBI (65,66), aSAH (67), and ICH (68). In addition, as will be further elaborated, a knowledge of the quality of pressure reactivity can potentially inform treatment decisions for intracranial hypertension based on the physiology outlined earlier. There is no bedside gold standard for assessing pressure autoregulation, and methods are often distinguished as "static" vs. "dynamic" (69). Static methods are based on the pharmacological manipulation of MAP and the observation of the effect on the direct measurement of CBF, CBF surrogates (eg, TCD FV (70), and brain tissue oxygenation (71) or ICP. Lassen, who originally used static methodology to construct the classic autoregulation curve, also showed that in chronically hypertensive individuals, the plateau of the autoregulatory curve is "shifted to the right," ie, toward higher MAPs (72). Static assessments attempt to identify the position on the curve at a given time point in a patient's course. The main disadvantages of static assessments are related to the inability to monitor changes over time and to the artificial nature of the testing, with the potential for interference and harm to patients by using vasoactive medications. Thus, dynamic changes in pressure reactivity related to spontaneous hemodynamic fluctuations have been employed for real-time monitoring.

Brain-injured critically ill patients under mechanical ventilation exhibit slow (20–200 second) ABP variations, leading to quantifiable cerebrovascular vasomotor responses (73,74). Czosnyka et al studied 83 severe TBI patients using an in-house software analysis of online physiological data to collect and calculate time-averaged values of ICP, ABP, CPP, and the middle cerebral artery FV; the authors used waveform time integration (average values of 256 consecutive samples) for 5-second intervals. A linear (Pearson's) moving correlation coefficient between 40 past consecutive 5-second averages of ICP and ABP, designated as PRx, was computed. Computations were repeated with a moving window every 5 seconds (66); current standards for computing PRx in long-term monitoring are slightly altered to a moving correlation coefficient between 30 values of consecutive 10-second ABP and ICP averages. A positive PRx signifies a positive gradient of the regression line between the slow components of ABP and ICP, indicating a passive nonreactive behavior of the vascular bed. A negative value of PRx reflects a normally reactive vascular bed, with ABP waves provoking inversely correlated waves in ICP (Figure 2.3). Because the correlation coefficient has a standardized value (range, −1 to +1), PRx provides a convenient index suitable for comparison between patients. A positive PRx correlated significantly with high ICP, a low-admission GCS score, and a poor outcome at 6 months after injury. The correlation between PRx and a TCD-derived index of autoregulation was highly significant (65).

PRx may be presented and analyzed as a time-dependent variable, responding to dynamic events such as ICP plateau waves or incidents of arterial

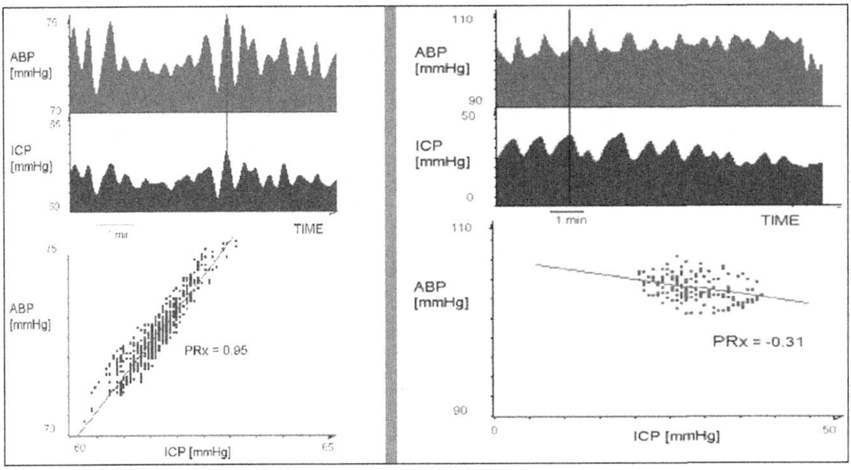

FIGURE 2.3 Pressure-reactivity index. The PRx is a Pearson's correlation coefficient between the waveforms of arterial blood pressure (ABP) and intracranial pressure (ICP).

hypotension, hypertension, or refractory intracranial hypertension. PRx has been validated against a PET-derived, static measure of autoregulation (static rate of autoregulation [$SROR_{PET}$]) (75). PRx and $SROR_{PET}$ were shown to correlate closely under conditions of disturbed pressure autoregulation (high PRx and low $SROR_{PET}$); the correlation was not as good for conditions of preserved reactivity (low PRx). This could be related to the limited precision of PET measurements in the face of minor or relatively stable CBF. The relationship of PRx with CBF and the cerebral metabolic rate for oxygen ($CMRO_2$) was explored in a group of 22 severe TBI patients (76). An inverse relationship between PRx and the $CMRO_2$ was found; the data relating the oxygen extraction fraction (OEF) and PRx followed a quadratic function with disturbed PRx for both low and high OEF. Absolute CBF did not correlate with PRx.

Compromised pressure-flow autoregulation, cerebral dysoxia, and metabolic failure are all features of severe TBI and seem to be related at different levels, yet we currently lack a satisfactory mechanistic model that links them. In an effort to explore these complex relationships, we recently performed a systematic review of multimodality monitoring (PRx, $PbtO_2$, and lactate to pyruvate ratio [LPR]), including 32 observational studies and two RCTs with a total of 1161 patient observations (77). Although the overall quality of evidence was moderate and several methodological biases were found, our interpretation of this literature suggests that the knowledge of the status of pressure autoregulation is essential not only to optimize CPP but to inform the approach and interventions targeted to $PbtO_2$ and LPR. Pressure reactivity could be the first step in approaching the relations among CBF, oxygen delivery/demand, and cellular metabolism.

In 2002 Steiner et al published a landmark study on the use of PRx as a means of identifying patient-specific CPPopt using long-term ICP/ABP monitoring in patients with severe TBI (78). This was a retrospective analysis of data from 114 consecutive TBI patients receiving intensive care and continuous multi-modality monitoring at Addenbrooke's Hospital, Cambridge, United Kingdom. CPPopt was defined as the CPP range (bins of 5 mmHg) corresponding to the lowest PRx value observed (the lower or more negative the PRx, the better the preserved pressure reactivity is considered to be). Then, the difference between actual mean CPP and CPPopt was calculated and shown to significantly correlate with 6-month outcome; outcome correlated with this difference both for patients who were managed on average below CPPopt and for patients whose mean CPP was above CPPopt. This finding enforced the concept of inappropriate perfusion pressures (on both sides of the spectrum) and their impact on clinical outcomes. Another important aspect is the demonstration of the dynamic nature of pressure autoregulation across and within patients, pointing against an "all or nothing" phenomenon and providing a strong physiological rationale for individualizing therapy. An important methodological limitation of this study was the fact that despite successfully obtaining CPPopt for the majority of patients, it was impossible to identify CPPopt for 40% of the cohort. The authors proposed a number of hypotheses for this failure, including a CPPopt lying outside the studied range, an inadequate time window and/or inadequate data points, and disturbed pressure reactivity for a different etiology than inappropriate CPP. Finally, Steiner et al proposed an algorithmic approach in identifying CPPopt, setting the stage for a PRx-targeted prospective trial.

More recently, Aries et al conducted a retrospective analysis of prospectively collected, long-term monitoring data of ICP and ABP in TBI patients using the ICM+ software (www.neurosurg.cam.ac.uk/icmplus) (79). The algorithm has been improved, incorporating an automatic U-shape curve fitting with a 4-hour-long moving window (Figure 2.4). CPPopt could be continuously calculated more than 80% of the time and presented as a dynamically changing variable. Continuous metrics of the distance between CPPopt and observed CPP related to patient outcome. For CPP too low in comparison to CPPopt, the mortality rate dramatically increased, and for CPP too high, the

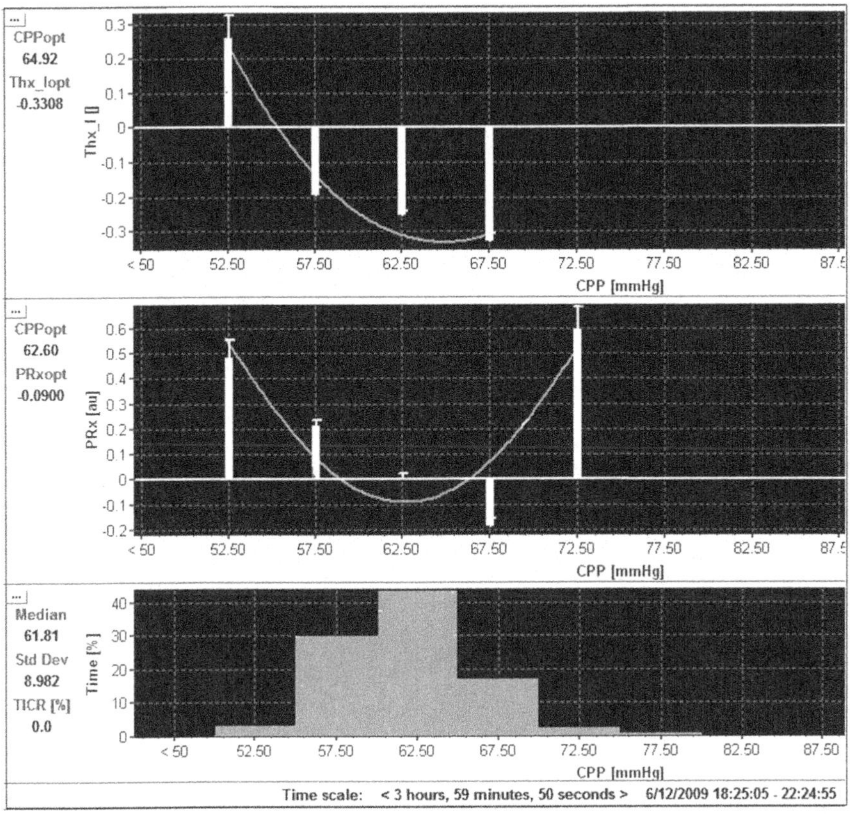

FIGURE 2.4 Cerebral perfusion pressure optimal curves based on 4-hour moving time windows.

incidence of severe disability increased. Favorable outcome reached its peak when CPP was maintained close to CPPopt. The value of PRx has also been demonstrated in a group of TBI pediatric patients, where it was significantly associated with survival (80). Pressure reactivity was found to improve with increasing CPP, and PRx was CPP dependent. PRx could play a role in helping to determine not only patient-specific but also age-specific CPPopt targets.

PRx was also recently used to define patient-specific ICP thresholds in patients with severe TBI (81). ICP "doses" were calculated based on three different thresholds, one based on PRx (patient specific) and the other two based on conventional thresholds of 20 and 25 mmHg. Doses based on PRx were stronger predictors of mortality than those calculated based on the standard generic thresholds. This finding further highlights the impact of intracranial hypertension, specifically in the presence of disturbed pressure reactivity, on clinical outcome and further supports the idea that individualized ICP/CPP thresholds should be sought. The concept of individualized CPPopt-guided therapy has not yet been prospectively tested in a randomized controlled manner; efforts are underway for a multicenter trial testing the CPPopt approach.

The Estimation of Cerebral Compliance Based on Intracranial Pressure Waveforms and Relevance to External Ventricular Drain Weaning

The ICP pulse waveform has three distinct harmonics that are related to physiological parameters (Figure 2.5). The first peak (P1), the "percussive" wave, is due to arterial pressure being transmitted from the choroid plexus to the ventricle. It is sharply peaked and fairly consistent in amplitude. The second wave (P2), often called the "tidal" wave, is thought to be due to brain tissue compliance. It is variable, indicates cerebral compliance, and generally increases in amplitude as compliance decreases. P3 is due to the closure of the aortic valve and therefore represents the dicrotic notch (12). It is often mentioned that in the presence of a larger P2 component, and despite acceptable mean ICP values, EVD weaning should be withheld. We are not aware of any empirical data confirming this warning.

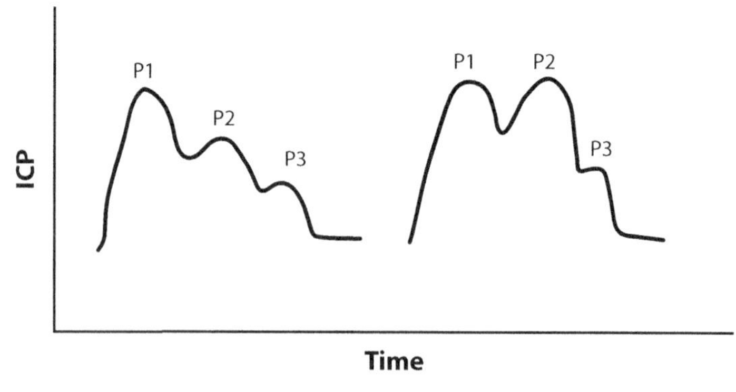

FIGURE 2.5 Intracranial pressure (ICP) by time graph (untitled). ICP waveforms showing the normal morphology on the left, and increased P2 wave amplitude suggesting poor intracranial compliance on the right.

Actual brain compliance is a rather complex physiologic entity. Czosnyka and Citerio recently reviewed it as a sum (it is not certain whether it is an algebraic sum) of three compliances:

$$\text{C brain} = \text{C venous pool (ICP, Pss, CVP)} + \text{C CSF pool (ICP, CVP, P0)} + \text{C arterial pool (CPP)},$$

where Pss is the sagittal sinus pressure, CVP is the central venous pressure, and P0 is the ICP reference pressure (82).

This formula hypothetically shows that the resulting brain compliance is a nonlinear function of many compartmental pressures, making direct measurements theoretically and technically difficult. An alternative way to assess the cerebrospinal pressure-volume relationship is via the slope of the amplitude-pressure regression, or RAP index (the correlation coefficient between slow changes in AMP and mean ICP) (83). The AMP is equivalent to a pressure-volume response measured with an unknown volume load, ie, brain fraction of heart stroke volume. The AMP/ICP regression slope is proportional to brain elasticity multiplied by the same stroke volume. The RAP index shows where the craniospinal "working point" is placed on the pressure-volume curve (on the linear part, exponential part, or above the "critical ICP"). The RAP index has not been studied in the setting of EVD weaning.

External ventricular drain weaning strategies

The optimal time to remove an EVD is when it has either fulfilled or failed the reason it was inserted in the first place. If it was placed for purely ICP monitoring reasons, then clinical improvement and/or stable ICP readings for 48 to 72 hours would indicate removal. If it was placed for CSF/blood diversion, as in the case of IVH, removal is indicated once the blood has cleared, and the hydrocephalus has resolved. Weaning strategy differs among protocols, institutions, and clinicians. Traditionally, once the primary reason for placement is resolving, the EVD is "raised" stepwise and eventually clamped before removal. The patient's clinical picture, hourly/daily CSF output, mean ICP readings, waveform morphology, and CT appearance are all taken into account. A common strategy is to raise the EVD by a height of 5 mmHg (7 cm H_2O) every 12 to 24 hours. Another general rule of thumb is that once the drain is at a level greater than 10 mmHg (13 cm H_2O), the continuation of EVD weaning should only be considered with a daily CSF output of less than 250 mL. Once the level has reached the 20 mmHg mark without complications, the EVD can be clamped. Often, the patient remains "clamped" for 24 hours before a CT head is performed to confirm no dilation of the ventricular system before removal.

Klopfenstein et al performed a randomized trial in aSAH of the conventional approach described earlier vs. "rapid weaning" of EVDs (84); 41 patients were randomized to the rapidly weaned group, and 40 were randomized to the gradually weaned group. The two groups were well matched. Rapid weaning was defined as occurring within 24 hours with immediate closure of the EVD. All patients in whom EVD weaning failed underwent shunt placement. Rates of shunt implantation, days in the intensive care unit (ICU), and the overall duration of hospitalization were compared. No significant difference existed in rates of shunt implantation between the rapidly weaned (63.4%) and the gradually weaned (62.5%) groups. Nevertheless, the length of stay for patients in the gradually weaned group increased significantly (a mean of 2.8 and 2.4 more days in the ICU and in the hospital, respectively). The fact that individual patient-specific and pathology-specific differences determine responses to freedom from EVD dependency should be considered, and longer periods of EVD insertion may, on occasion, eliminate the need for a shunt procedure altogether.

In regard to the timing of converting from a failed EVD to a ventriculoperitoneal shunt (VPS), another recent study showed that no delay is necessary because of IVH or proteinaceous CSF in the setting of aSAH (85). Finally, a recent study assessed the prediction for VPS placement in association with the type of EVD-weaning failure. A significant association with failure was due to clinical changes, whereas weaning failure due to elevated ICP or radiographic changes was not predictive (86).

External ventricular drain malfunction, occlusion, and ventricular collapse

Ventricular catheter displacement and blockage are not uncommon. Blood clots or fibrin deposits can obliterate the small holes at the tip of the catheter, and the catheter can become displaced so that part or all of its tip sits in the brain parenchyma rather than in the ventricle. Poor CSF drainage and ICP waveform are indications of either misplacement or obstruction. If it happens soon after insertion, brain imaging should be considered.

If a catheter obstruction is suspected (particularly in the presence of a clot or debris in the tubing), gentle flushing with sterile, preservative-free saline can often restore the catheter patency; the procedure should be performed with the maximum attention to asepsis, as repeated manipulations of the EVD system are associated with a higher incidence of central nervous system infections (13).

The overdrainage of CSF may cause collapse of the lateral ventricles, leading to contact between the walls of the lateral ventricle and the ventricular catheter and causing obstruction. Overdrainage may also predispose patients to developing a subdural hematoma or hygroma. The incidence of these complications varies in different studies and populations. A study in pediatric patients, where an EVD was placed in the settings of TBI, hydrocephalus, or due to VPS failure, found that complications occurred in 26% of EVD insertions and included infection (9.4%), misplacement (6.3%), hemorrhage (4.2%), obstruction (3.1%), and malfunction (3.1%).

Acknowledgement

We would like to thank and acknowledge Professor Marek Czosnyka from the Department of Clinical Neurosciences, University of Cambridge, United Kingdom, for kindly providing Figures 2.1 through 2.4.

Disclaimer

The authors have no conflicts of interest in relation to this work. This is an invited review. No funding has been received for this work.

References

1. Bratton SL, Chestnut RM, Ghajar J, et al. Guidelines for the management of severe traumatic brain injury. Indications for intracranial pressure monitoring. *J Neurotrauma*. May 2007;24(suppl 1):S-37–S-44.
2. Stocchetti N, Picetti E, Berardino M, et al. Clinical applications of intracranial pressure monitoring in traumatic brain injury: report of the Milan consensus conference. *Acta Neurochir* (Vienna). 2014;156(8):1615–1622.
3. Helbok R, Olson DM, Le Roux PD, et al. Participants in the International Multidisciplinary Consensus Conference on Multimodality Monitoring. Intracranial pressure and cerebral perfusion pressure monitoring in non-TBI patients: special considerations. *Neurocrit Care*. December 2014;21(suppl 2):85–94.
4. Heuer GG, Smith MJ, Elliott JP, et al. Relationship between intracranial pressure and other clinical variables in patients with aneurysmal subarachnoid hemorrhage. *J Neurosurg*. 2004;101:408–416.
5. Ryttlefors M, Howells T, Nilsson P, et al. Secondary insults in subarachnoid hemorrhage: occurrence and impact on outcome and clinical deterioration. *Neurosurgery*. 2007;61: 704–714(discussion):714–715.
6. Citerio G, Gaini SM, Tomei G, et al. Management of 350 aneurysmal subarachnoid hemorrhages in 22 italian neurosurgical centers. *Intensive Care Med*. 2007;33:1580–1586.
7. Adams RE, Diringer MN. Response to external ventricular drainage in spontaneous intracerebral hemorrhage with hydrocephalus. *Neurology*. 1998;50:519–523.

8. Coplin WM, Vinas FC, Agris JM, et al. A cohort study of the safety and feasibility of intraventricular urokinase for nonaneurysmal spontaneous intraventricular hemorrhage. *Stroke.* 1998;29:1573–1579.

9. Ziai WC, Melnychuk E, Thompson CB, et al. Occurrence and impact of intracranial pressure elevation during treatment of severe intraventricular hemorrhage. *Crit Care Med.* 2012;40:1601–1608.

10. Zweifel C, Czosnyka M, Carrera E, et al. Reliability of the blood flow velocity pulsatility index for assessment of intracranial and cerebral perfusion pressures in head-injured patients. *Neurosurgery.* 2012;71(4):853–861.

11. Sekhon MS, Griesdale DE, Robba C, et al. Optic nerve sheath diameter on computed tomography is correlated with simultaneously measured intracranial pressure in patients with severe traumatic brain injury. *Intensive Care Med.* 2014;40(9):1267–1274.

12. Citerio G, Andrews PJ. Intracranial pressure. Part two: clinical applications and technology. *Intensive Care Med.* 2004;30(10):1882–1885.

13. Lavinio A, Menon DK. Intracranial pressure: why we monitor it, how to monitor it, what to do with the number and what's the future? *Curr Opin Anaesthesiol.* 2011;24(2): 117–123.

14. Piek J, Raes P. Pressure-controlled drainage of cerebrospinal fluid: clinical experience with a new type of ventricular catheter (Ventcontrol MTC) and an integrated Piezo-resistive sensor at its tip: technical note. *Neurosurgery.* 1996;38:216–218.

15. Flibotte JJ, Lee KE, Koroshetz WJ, et al. Continuous antibiotic prophylaxis and cerebral spinal fluid infection in patients with intracranial pressure monitors. *Neurocrit Care.* 2004;1: 61–68.

16. Lozier AP, Sciacca RR, Romagnoli MF, et al. Ventriculostomy related infections: a critical review of the literature. *Neurosurgery.* 2008;62(suppl 2):688–700.

17. Chatzi M, Karvouniaris M, Makris D, et al. Bundle of measures for external cerebral ventricular drainage-associated ventriculitis. *Crit Care Med.* 2014;42(1):66–73.

18. Zabramski JM, Whiting D, Darouiche RO, et al. Efficacy of antimicrobial impregnated external ventricular drain catheters: a prospective, randomized, controlled trial. *J Neurosurg.* 2003;98:725–730.

19. Fichtner J, Guresir E, Seifert V, et al. Efficacy of silver-bearing external ventricular drainage catheters: a retrospective analysis. *J Neurosurg.* 2010;112:840–846.

20. Harrop JS, Sharan AD, Ratliff J, et al. Impact of a standardized protocol and antibiotic-impregnated catheters on ventriculostomy infection rates in cerebrovascular patients. *Neurosurgery.* 2010;67(1):187–191.

21. Hetem DJ, Woerdeman PA, Bonten MJ, et al. Relationship between bacterial colonization of external cerebrospinal fluid drains and secondary meningitis: a retrospective analysis of an 8-year period. *J Neurosurg.* 2010;113:1309–1313.

22. Piper I, Barnes A, Smith D, et al. The Camino intracranial pressure sensor: is it optimal technology? An internal audit with a review of current intracranial pressure monitoring technologies. *Neurosurgery.* 2001;49:1158–1164.

23. Chambers IR, Siddique MS, Banister K, et al. Clinical comparison of the Spiegelberg parenchymal transducer and ventricular fluid pressure. *J Neurol Neurosurg Psychiatry.* 2001;71: 383–385.

24. Czosnyka M, Czosnyka Z, Pickard JD. Laboratory testing of three intracranial pressure microtransducers: technical report. *Neurosurgery.* 1996;38:219–224.

25. Czosnyka M, Pickard JD. Monitoring and interpretation of intracranial pressure. *J Neurol Neurosurg Psychiatry* [review]. 2004;75(6):813–821.

26. Hutchinson PJ, Hutchinson DB, Barr RH, et al. A new cranial access device for cerebral monitoring. *Br J Neurosurg*. 2000;14:46–48.

27. Wolfla CE, Luerssen TG, Bowman RM, et al. Brain tissue pressure gradients created by expanding frontal epidural mass lesion. *J Neurosurg*. 1996;84:642–647.

28. Frank JI. Large hemispheric infarction, deterioration, and intracranial pressure. *Neurology*. 1995;45(7):1286–1290.

29. Czosnyka M, Whitehouse H, Smielewski P, et al. Testing of cerebrospinal compensatory reserve in shunted and non-shunted patients: a guide to interpretation based on an observational study. *J Neurol Neurosurg Psychiatry*. 1996;60:549–558.

30. Gjerris F, Brogesen SE. Pathophysiology of CSF circulation. In: Crockard A, Hayward A, Hoff JT, eds. *Neurosurgery: The Scientific Basis of Clinical Practice*. Oxford: Blackwell Scientific; 1992:146–174.

31. Pickard JD, Teasdale G, Matherson M, et al. Intraventricular pressure waves—the best predictive test for shunting in normal pressure hydrocephalus. In: Shulman K, Marmarou A, Miller JD, Becker DP, Hochwold GM, Brock M, eds. *Intracranial Pressure IV*. Berlin: Springer-Verlag; 1980:498–500.

32. Newell DW, Aaslid R, Stross R, et al. The relationship of blood flow velocity fluctuations to intracranial pressure B waves. *J Neurosurg*. 1992;76:415–421.

33. Owler BK, Fong KC, Czosnyka Z. Importance of ICP monitoring in the investigation of CSF circulation disorders. *Br J Neurosurg*. 2001;15(5):439–440.

34. Li LM, Timofeev I, Czosnyka M, et al. Review article: the surgical approach to the management of increased intracranial pressure after traumatic brain injury. *Anesth Analg*. 2010;111(3):736–748.

35. Servadei F, Picetti E. Intracranial pressure monitoring and outcome in traumatic brain injury: the probe does matter? *World Neurosurg* [e-pub ahead of print]. February 5, 2015.

36. Chesnut R, Videtta W, Vespa P, et al. Participants in the International Multidisciplinary Consensus Conference on Multimodality Monitoring. Intracranial pressure monitoring: fundamental considerations and rationale for monitoring. *Neurocrit Care*. December 2014;21(suppl 2):64–84.

37. Sahuquillo J, Poca M-A, Arribas M, et al. Interhemispheric supratentorial intracranial pressure gradients in head-injured patients: are they clinically important? *J Neurosurg*. 1999; 90(1):16–26.

38. Exo J, Kochanek PM, Adelson PD, et al. Intracranial pressure-monitoring systems in children with traumatic brain injury: combining therapeutic and diagnostic tools. *Pediatr Crit Care Med*. 2011;12(5):560–565.

39. Soehle M, Chatfield DA, Czosnyka M, et al. Predictive value of initial clinical status, intracranial pressure and transcranial Doppler pulsatility after subarachnoid haemorrhage. *Acta Neurochir* (Vienna). 2007;149(6):575–583.

40. Phillips SB, Gates M, Krishnamurthy S. Strategic placement of bedside ventriculostomies using ultrasound image guidance: report of three cases. *Neurocrit Care*. 2012;17(2): 255–259.

41. Jakola AS, Reinertsen I, Selbekk T, et al. Three-dimensional ultrasound-guided placement of ventricular catheters. *World Neurosurg*. 2014;82(3–4):536.e5–9.

42. Binz DD, Toussaint LG III, Friedman JA. Hemorrhagic complications of ventriculostomy placement: a meta-analysis. *Neurocrit Care*. 2009;10(2):253–256.

43. Matevosyan K, Madden C, Barnett SL, et al. Coagulation factor levels in neurosurgical patients with mild prolongation of prothrombin time: effect on plasma transfusion therapy. *J Neurosurg*. 2010;114:3–7.

44. Bauer DF, McGwin G Jr, Melton SM, et al. The relationship between INR and development of hemorrhage with placement of ventriculostomy. *J Trauma*. 2011;70(5):1112–1117.

45. Martinez-Manas RM, Santamarta D, de Campos JM, et al. Camino intracranial pressure monitor: prospective study of accuracy and complications. *J Neurol Neurosurg Psychiatry*. 2000;69:82–86.

46. Stocchetti N, Maas AI. Traumatic intracranial hypertension. *N Engl J Med*. 2014; 371(10):972.

47. Lozier AP, Sciacca RR, Romagnoli MF, et al. Ventriculostomy-related infections: a critical review of the literature. *Neurosurgery*. 2002;51:170–181.

48. Beer R, Pfausler B, Schmutzhard E. Infectious intracranial complications in the neuro-ICU patient population. *Curr Opin Crit Care*. 2010;16(2):117–122.

49. Koskinen LO, Grayson D, Olivecrona M. The complications and the position of the Codman MicroSensor™ ICP device: an analysis of 549 patients and 650 sensors. *Acta Neurochir* (Vienna). 2013;155(11):2141–2148.

50. Lassen NA. Cerebral blood flow and oxygen consumption in man. *Physiol Rev*. 1959;39:183–238.

51. Rosner MJ, Coley IB. Cerebral perfusion pressure, intracranial pressure, and head elevation. *J Neurosurg Anesthesiol*. 1986;65:636–641.

52. Kosty JA, Leroux PD, Levine J, et al. Brief report: a comparison of clinical and research practices in measuring cerebral perfusion pressure: a literature review and practitioner survey. *Anesth Analg*. 2013;117(3):694–698.

53. Olson DM, Batjer HH, Abdulkadir K, et al. Measuring and monitoring ICP in neurocritical care: results from a national practice survey. *Neurocrit Care*. 2014;20(1):15–20.

54. Davson H, Hollingsworth G, Segal MB. The mechanism of drainage of the cerebrospinal fluid. *Brain*. 1970;93:665–678.

55. Lundberg N. Continuous recording and control of ventricular fluid pressure in neurosurgical practice. *Acta Psychiatr Neurol Scand*. 1960;36(suppl 149):1–193.

56. Andrews PJ, Citerio G. Intracranial pressure. Part one: historical overview and basic concepts. *Intensive Care Med*. 2004;30(9):1730–1733.

57. Czosnyka M, Smielewski P, Piechnik S, et al. Hemodynamic characterization of intracranial pressure plateau waves in head-injury patients. *J Neurosurg*. 1999;91(1):11–19.

58. Czosnyka M, Smielewski P, Timofeev I, et al. Intracranial pressure: more than a number. *Neurosurg Focus*. 2007;22(5):E10.

59. Avezaat CJ, van Eijndhoven JH, Wyper DJ. Cerebrospinal fluid pulse pressure and intra- cranial volume-pressure relationships. *J Neurol Neurosurg Psychiatry*. 1979;42:687–700.

60. Eide PK, Sorteberg W. Association among intracranial compliance, intracranial pulse pressure amplitude and intracranial pressure in patients with intracranial bleeds. *Neurol Res*. 2007;29:798–802.

61. Radolovich DK, Aries MJ, Castellani G, et al. Pulsatile intracranial pressure and cerebral autoregulation after traumatic brain injury. *Neurocrit Care*. 2011;15(3):379–386.

62. Eide PK, Sorteberg A, Bentsen G, et al. Pressure-derived versus pressure wave amplitude-derived indices of cerebrovascular pressure reactivity in relation to early clinical state and 12-month outcome following aneurysmal subarachnoid hemorrhage. *J Neurosurg*. 2012;116(5):961–971.

63. Eide PK, Bentsen G, Sorteberg AG, et al. A randomized and blinded single-center trial comparing the effect of intracranial pressure and intracranial pressure wave amplitude-guided intensive care management on early clinical state and 12-month outcome in patients with aneurysmal subarachnoid hemorrhage. *Neurosurgery*. 2011;69(5):1105–1115.

64. Lazaridis C, Smielewski P, Steiner LA, et al. Optimal cerebral perfusion pressure: are we ready for it? *Neurol Res.* 2013;35(2):138–148.

65. Czosnyka M, Smielewski P, Kirkpatrick P, et al. Monitoring of cerebral autoregulation in head injured patients. *Stroke.* 1996;27(10):1829–1834.

66. Czosnyka M, Smielewski P, Kirkpatrick P, et al. Continuous assessment of the cerebral vasomotor reactivity in head injury. *Neurosurgery.* 1997;41(1):11–17;(discussion):17–19.

67. Jaeger M, Schuhmann MU, Soehle M, et al. Continuous monitoring of cerebrovascular autoregulation after subarachnoid hemorrhage by brain tissue oxygen pressure reactivity and its relation to delayed cerebral infarction. *Stroke.* 2007;38:981–986.

68. Diedler J, Sykora M, Rupp A, et al. Impaired cerebral vasomotor activity in spontaneous intracerebral hemorrhage. *Stroke.* 2009;40:815–819.

69. Panerai RB. Assessment of cerebral pressure autoregulation in humans—a review of measurement methods [review]. *Physiol Meas.* 1998;19(3):305–338.

70. Tiecks FP, Lam AM, Aaslid R, et al. Comparison of static and dynamic cerebral autoregulation measurements. *Stroke.* 1995;26(6):1014–1019.

71. Jaeger M, Schuhmann MU, Soehle M, et al. Continuous monitoring of cerebrovascular autoregulation after subarachnoid hemorrhage by brain tissue oxygen pressure reactivity and its relation to delayed cerebral infarction. *Stroke.* 2007;38:981–986.

72. Strandgaard S, Olesen J, Skinhoj E, et al. Autoregulation of brain circulation in severe arterial hypertension. *Br Med J.* 1973;1(5852):507–510.

73. Rosner MJ, Becker DP. Origin and evolution of plateau waves. Experimental observations and a theoretical model. *J Neurosurg.* 1984;60:312–324.

74. Aaslid R, Lindegaard KF, Sorteberg W, et al. Cerebral autoregulation dynamics in humans. *Stroke.* 1989;20(1):45–52.

75. Steiner LA, Coles JP, Johnston AJ, et al. Assessment of cerebrovascular autoregulation in head-injured patients: a validation study. *Stroke.* 2003;34(10):2404–2409.

76. Steiner LA, Coles JP, Czosnyka M, et al. Cerebrovascular pressure reactivity is related to global cerebral oxygen metabolism after head injury. *J Neurol Neurosurg Psychiatry.* 2003;74(6):765–770.

77. Lazaridis C, Andrews CM. Brain tissue oxygenation, lactate-pyruvate ratio, and cerebrovascular pressure reactivity monitoring in severe traumatic brain injury: systematic review and viewpoint. *Neurocrit Care.* 2014;21(2):345–355.

78. Steiner LA, Czosnyka M, Piechnik SK, et al. Continuous monitoring of cerebrovascular pressure reactivity allows determination of optimal cerebral perfusion pressure in patients with traumatic brain injury. *Crit Care Med.* 2002;30(4):733–738.

79. Aries MJ, Czosnyka M, Budohoski KP, et al. Continuous monitoring of cerebrovascular reactivity using pulse waveform of intracranial pressure. *Neurocrit Care.* 2012;17(1):67–76.

80. Brady KM, Shaffner DH, Lee JK, et al. Continuous monitoring of cerebrovascular pressure reactivity after traumatic brain injury in children. *Pediatrics.* 2009;124(6):e1205–1212.

81. Lazaridis C, DeSantis SM, Smielewski P, et al. Patient-specific thresholds of intracranial pressure in severe traumatic brain injury. *J Neurosurg.* 2014;120(4):893–900.

82. Czosnyka M, Citerio G. Brain compliance: the old story with a new "et cetera." *Intensive Care Med.* 2012;38(6):925–927.

83. Czosnyka M, Guazzo E, Whitehouse M, et al. Significance of intracranial pressure waveform analysis after head injury. *Acta Neurochir* (Vienna). 1996;138:531–541;(discussion):541–542.

84. Klopfenstein JD, Kim LJ, Feiz-Erfan I, et al. Comparison of rapid and gradual weaning from external ventricular drainage in patients with aneurysmal subarachnoid hemorrhage: a prospective randomized trial. *J Neurosurg.* 2004;100(2):225–229.

85. Kang DH, Park J, Park SH, et al. Early ventriculoperitoneal shunt placement after severe aneurysmal subarachnoid hemorrhage: role of intraventricular hemorrhage and shunt function. *Neurosurgery*. 2010;66(5):904–909.

86. Lewis A, Taylor Kimberly W. Prediction of ventriculoperitoneal shunt placement based on type of failure during external ventricular drain wean. *Clin Neurol Neurosurg*. October 2014;125:109–113.

3

Controversies in Intracranial Pressure Monitoring

Kristine H. O'Phelan
Starane A. I. Shepherd
Indira DeJesus-Alvelo

In this chapter we will discuss several recent controversies about how and when to monitor intracranial pressure (ICP). In general, level 1 evidence supporting ICP monitoring in acute brain injury is sparse. We will discuss in some detail the results of the recently published Benchmark Evidence from South American Trials: Treatment of Intracranial Pressure (BEST TRIP) trial, which provides what little high-quality data we have for ICP monitoring in traumatic brain injury (TBI) but has many limitations nonetheless. This trial has served to focus our attention on how we use monitoring and whether we are leveraging the information adequately to help our patients. We will discuss the potential paradigm shifts in our management strategies that are developing in response to these data. We will also present data to support or refute the use of ICP monitoring in certain common types of acute brain injury, with a focus on different monitoring methods.

Is there a role for intracranial pressure monitoring after Benchmark Evidence from South American Trials: Treatment of Intracranial Pressure?

In 2012, Carney et al (1,2) published BEST TRIP, a prospective, randomized controlled trial to determine if monitoring ICP has an impact on mortality and neuropsychological functional outcomes in patients who survive TBI. This study was performed in six Latin American centers (four in Bolivia and two in

Ecuador) where ICP monitors are not consistently used as the standard of care in the management of patients with severe TBI. The study used a two-group parallel design, in which the intervention was not blinded. Between 2008 and 2011, 324 patients were enrolled. Inclusion criteria included an age older than 12 years, no foreign objects in the brain parenchyma, and a Glasgow Coma Scale (GCS) score of less than 8 (with a motor scale score of less than 5) within 24 hours of injury. Patients who had a neurological deterioration meeting this criteria within 48 hours of injury were also eligible. Further stratification and randomization were performed to compare patients younger and older than 40 years and patients with a GCS score of 3 to 5 vs. a score of 6 to 8. Data collected included pupillary function, GCS on arrival, the presence or absence of hypotensive episodes, hypoxia, and CT findings. The two treatment groups were Standard versus Intervention.

The Standard group received a treatment protocol based on the experience of local physicians but had no quantitative data. Empiric treatment was applied depending on the clinician's interpretations of neurological worsening or follow-up CT findings.

The Intervention group had an intraparenchymal ICP monitor placed. A standardized treatment protocol was applied when ICP was greater than 20 mmHg for more than 5 minutes, and failure to treat was defined as the inability to control the ICP within 20 minutes. ICP monitors were removed after 24 hours of ICP values less than 20 mmHg without any medical intervention.

This study found no significant differences in outcomes between the two groups except that the Standard group received more days of brain-specific treatments (3% normal saline and hyperventilation) than the Intervention group. Also, more barbiturates were administered, and higher rates of decubitus ulcers were reported in the Intervention group. This trial represents an important milestone in neurocritical care because it is a prospective, randomized study to address the issue of ICP monitoring. However, its limitations include a lack of documentation of secondary insults both in the prehospital phase as well as in the intensive care unit (ICU). Although the Intervention protocol included the rapid identification and treatment of elevated ICP, there is concern that this was not always provided to the Intervention group. Furthermore, far fewer resources are available in Latin America for aggressive postacute and rehabilitation care. This may have had a negative impact on patients in both the Standard and Intervention groups and may have been a stronger determinant of outcome than the treatments provided in the ICU.

Is this study going to change the current practice?

The most recent Guidelines for Management of Severe TBI (3) published in 2007 establish level II recommendations to place ICP monitors in patients with severe TBI (GCS score 3 to 8) with an abnormal CT (showing contusions, hematomas, swelling, herniation, or compressed basal cisterns). Level III recommendations support placement of an ICP monitor in patients with severe TBI and normal CT scans if two or more of these criteria are met: an age older than 40 years, unilateral or bilateral abnormal posturing, or a systolic blood pressure (BP) less than 90 mmHg upon admission. ICP has been well recognized as a strong predictor of outcome in severe TBI (4), and treatments based on established values thresholds have been recommended because of this fact. Elevated ICP can be the first sign of worsening intracranial pathology and surgical mass lesions, therefore detecting a rise in ICP intuitively may lead to earlier therapy.

It is important to determine if the BEST TRIP trial results can be generalized to other geographic regions and should influence our current guidelines. Prehospital care is now recognized to be as important as intrahospital care since prehospital hypotension (systolic BP less than 90 mmHg) is an independent predictor of poor outcome after severe TBI. In the BEST TRIP trial, the mean time from injury to arrival at the study center was approximately 3.1 hours. Unfortunately, this study contains inconsistent prehospital and early care documentation (5). It is likely that many patients enrolled in this study were hypotensive or hypoxic prior to arriving at the medical center. The influence of these insults may overcome any benefit that ICP monitoring in the ICU provides. One must also consider whether the patients enrolled in the BEST TRIP trial are as severely injured as the population that we identify and treat in North America and Europe. Perhaps the prehospital care available in the United States selects for more neurologically disabled patients to make it to the hospital? This remains a matter of debate and disagreement; however, the study's authors contend that "ICU demographics, treatment courses and short term (14 days) outcomes appear comparable to US and European situations" (6). This supports the "cautious interpretation" and generalization of the BEST TRIP trial results to low-, middle-, and high-income countries.

The fact that the Standard group received treatment for signs of elevated ICP even when an ICP monitor was not placed to quantitatively confirm abnormal pressures and/or treatment response must also be considered. Therefore, the more accurate question that this trial poses is whether it is better to treat ICP with or without a monitor, not whether ICP is important.

Perhaps the BEST TRIP trial challenges our complacency about ICP rather than a study of ICP-monitoring efficacy (7). This is an opportunity to change our traditional views and use ICP in a different way to individualize treatment based on directly observing and interpreting all the information obtained from multimodal monitoring (MMM). This offers the potential to target all mechanisms involved in secondary brain injury (SBI). MMM includes the evaluation of microvascular dysfunction and impaired glucose utilization as independent SBI factors that ICP or CPP abnormalities may or may not accompany. The identification, prevention, and management of SBI is the cornerstone of modern TBI care. Because of the complexity and heterogeneity of TBI pathophysiology, understanding what is happening in each patient is crucial.

As expected, authors from Latin America also had something to say about the BEST TRIP trial. Murillo-Cabezas and Godoy (8) from Argentina make the point of interpreting this trial not as a demonstration of the futility of ICP monitoring but as evidence of the need to redefine how to use ICP monitoring values to guide treatment. This also illustrates the need to establish a valid, reliable, accurate noninvasive technique to detect signs of intracranial hypertension when the invasive alternative is not readily available. This technique was novel for many of the physicians involved in this study. The inevitable learning curve with regard to ICP monitor placement and the correct interpretation and timely response to abnormal values is another controversial topic and should be considered when interpreting these trial results. Additionally, the interobserver variability among physicians reading and interpreting images was not formally analyzed and considered. This may also lead to confounded results.

The BEST TRIP trial provides additional evidence that ICP monitoring will never make the difference by itself. ICP values must be accurately interpreted and responded to, leading to individualized treatment that can influence a patient's outcome (6,8).

THRESHOLDS FOR INTRACRANIAL PRESSURE THERAPY

Is 20 mmHg a magic number?

Level 1 evidence to support the threshold value of 20 mmHg for determination of an elevated ICP is lacking. However, this value is well entrenched in neurocritical care. The relationship between elevations of ICP and mortality after TBI was elucidated by data collected in the 1960s by Jennett in Glasgow (9). In fact, one of the initial goals and objectives of the National Traumatic

Coma Data Bank, which started collecting data in 1979, was to better understand the utility of measuring ICP after TBI. By the time the first publication of the National Traumatic Coma Data Bank (10) was published in 1981, the value of 20 mmHg had been established in its data collection tools to indicate the presence of elevated ICP. Subsequent researchers adopted this and incorporated it into the guidelines for managing TBI in Europe and the United States (3). Solid physiological data does support the threshold of 20 mmHg. In a paper published in 1984, Rosner and Becker reported a study that carefully measured plateau waves in injured cats (11). Plateau waves are significant elevations of ICP to levels of 50 to 100 mmHg lasting from 3 to 30 minutes (12). They are characterized by spontaneous and acute elevations above a moderately raised baseline. This baseline was found to be 15 to 25 mmHg with a mean of 21 mmHg.

After 30 years of TBI research in this tradition, we come to the data provided by the recent BEST TRIP trial discussed earlier. This study's inability to demonstrate that monitoring ICP and treating elevations greater than 20 mmHg improve the 6-month outcome after TBI has caused many to question previously accepted assumptions. This is likely a good thing. Our current algorithms are linear, with a specific ICP value as the target. This is commonly known as a *stepwise approach* (Table 3.1). This approach assumes that the pathophysiology of head injuries across patients is similar and that each patient will

TABLE 3.1 A "stepwise" approach to intracranial pressure (ICP) management

Targets: CPP 60–70; ICP < 20; $PbtO_2$ >19; Temp <37C; CVP 6–10 Maintain CPP with fluids and pressors as needed	
Stage 1	Position: Head up 30–45° Sedation: Propofol, Analgesia: opiates Ventilation: pCO_2: 35–40 mmHg Temp: normothermia : 37.5°C CSF drainage
Stage 2	Osmotherapy
Stage 3	Neuromuscular Paralysis Mild Hyperventilation: pCO_2: 32–35 mmHg
Stage 4	Mild Hypothermia: @ 34–35° change sedative to benzodiazepine infusion
Stage 5	Decompressive Craniectomy
Stage 6	Metabolic suppression: Barbiturate sedation

Note: CPP, cerebral perfusion pressure; CSF, cerebral blood flow.

respond to an individual treatment in a predictable way. The main difference between patients is how far up the staircase one must climb (5). This is not likely to be far given the heterogeneity of human TBI.

So if ICP is not the target, perhaps it is a tool to understand the underlying pathophysiology and choose targets most likely to produce a beneficial effect. We do know that physiology is an important factor affecting the management of the developing brain. Cerebral perfusion pressure targets are age specific in pediatric TBI, and time spent below these targets increases short-term mortality considerably (13). In adults, cerebral compliance and autoregulation are dynamic processes that change over time after TBI. Specifically, older patients have worse compliance at higher ICP thresholds (14). Bedside examination can yield valuable information about brain compliance by considering the ICP response to usual stimulation such as turning, coughing, or suctioning. Thus, observed brain compliance understood through ICP monitoring can be used to determine a particular patient's need for more or less aggressive therapies.

How do you individualize treatments?

A number of "high-tech" strategies incorporate ICP to provide information about autoregulation and brain compliance. These methods are more quantitative and useful for research and for establishing therapeutic targets. The pressure reactivity index (PRx) (15), the relationship between mean arterial pressure (MAP) and ICP, is measured continuously over time in an individual patient. Thus, it can give information about the state of a particular patient at a particular time. Lazaridis et al published a study of 327 patients with severe TBI who underwent continuous ICP and MAP monitoring and the continuous calculation of PRx to demonstrate the optimal ICP threshold for each patient. The threshold values for ICP had a mean of 25 with an interquartile range of 20 to 32 and a standard deviation of 10 mmHg, meaning that many patients had threshold values considerably below and above the usual value of 20 mmHg (16). Additionally, they found that a patient's time spent above the calculated threshold correlated better with outcome at 6 months than did time spent above the traditional thresholds of 20 mmHg or 25 mmHg.

Another approach to choosing an individual ICP threshold is to consider ICP information in the context of other monitors. Many forms of monitoring the brain for disturbances of blood flow, electrophysiology, or metabolism are used in neurointensive care units. Some of these monitors provide information about the entire brain (electroencephalogram [EEG]), and some provide more regional information about blood flow (flowmetry) or metabolism (microdialysis). The information from different modalities of monitoring can be used together to determine the appropriate threshold for treating an elevated ICP.

Ultimately, the current controversies concerning ICP treatment thresholds serve to move neurocritical care toward more complex strategies using parallel approaches adjusted for individual patient characteristics. These approaches are inherently more flexible and dynamic and can be targeted to an individual patient's needs.

Intraventricular vs. intraparenchymal monitors—are intraventricular monitors better?

The 2007 Brain Trauma Foundation (BTF) guidelines also favor ventricular catheters connected to an external strain gauge as the "most accurate, low cost and reliable method of monitoring ICP." These catheters can be recalibrated in situ and allow fluid to drain as needed in patients with elevated ICP. However, complications, such as obstruction in fluid-coupled ventricular catheters causing malfunction and inaccurate values from improper leveling of the external transducer, can arise during their use. On the other hand, intraparenchymal monitors cannot be recalibrated during monitoring, may experience drift, and do not allow drainage of fluid if desired.

Interestingly, Vender et al (17) performed simultaneous intraventricular and parenchymal monitoring in order to have both a continuous pressure reading and continuous cerebrospinal fluid (CSF) drainage. They found that intraparenchymal monitor measurements were equally or more reliable when compared with ventriculostomy catheters. This prospective study was conducted with 11 patients who had severe closed TBI requiring no intracranial mass lesion evacuation. Intraparenchymal monitors may also have the advantage of lower rates of infectious and hemorrhagic complications.

EXTERNAL VENTRICULAR DRAIN STRATEGIES

What is the difference between an intermittent and a continuous external ventricular drain?

CSF drainage via an external ventricular drain (EVD) is considered the gold standard in situations of increased ICP as a result of TBI or subarachnoid hemorrhage (SAH). However, in the neurocritical and neurosurgical communities there remains clinical equipoise regarding the optimal CSF drainage strategy. CSF can be drained either intermittently or continuously. In the intermittent drainage strategy, which is more commonly used, ICP is continuously monitored, and the EVD is opened in response to sustained ICP elevation. For example, when ICP is above 20 mmHg for 5 minutes, the EVD is opened to release CSF and thereby lower ICP, as the Monro-Kellie doctrine explains. However, some physicians advocate for continuous CSF drainage. In this method, the EVD is left open and continuously drains CSF. The EVD is closed only when the physician wishes to accurately monitor ICP. For example, the EVD would be set to drain continuously at 15 mmHg and closed for 5 minutes every hour.

Proponents of continuous drainage assert that it may reduce the incidence of secondary injury in patients with TBI and SAH due to the increased removal of blood products and their metabolites and various inflammatory products. Shore et al used a prospective observational study to examine the effect of both drainage strategies on biochemical markers and ICP in CSF in a pediatric population. The authors demonstrated lower CSF concentrations of markers associated with neuronal injury in patients who were continuously drained, along with a lower mean ICP (18). However, it is unclear if the CSF concentration of biomarkers is representative of its interstitial concentration. Furthermore, this study did not assess morbidity or mortality as an outcome measure, so the association of these biomarkers with functional outcome remains unclear.

Is it possible to continuously drain cerebrospinal fluid while monitoring intracranial pressure?

While the EVD system is set to continuously drain, ICP cannot be measured because such measurement depends on a closed system. Opponents of continuous drainage cite this disadvantage. Some argue that if the EVD is continuously left open, an ICP crisis may go undetected and undertreated. To address this issue, some institutions place an intraparenchymal (IP) monitor adjacent to the EVD. This provides a corresponding ICP value as the EVD is draining. A study conducted with a pediatric TBI population compared ICP readings between an IP monitor and the EVD and showed a high correlation between these values. The authors suggested that this two-monitor system might be useful when using continuous CSF drainage as a therapeutic option (19). It should be noted that this might not accurately represent ICP in all cases, as the EVD measures a sum of pressures, while the IP monitor evaluates the parenchymal pressure at its tip. This pressure reading may differ from location to location, depending on distance from the injury or mass lesion (20). A new device can now monitor ICP while continuously draining CSF by integrating pressure transducers into the ventricular catheter; however, it has not been adopted for widespread use, and studies comparing its use to the standard EVD have yet to be performed (21).

Does continuous cerebrospinal fluid drainage increase the risk of overdrainage?

The overdrainage of CSF is a valid concern. Overdrainage can occur during episodes of patient coughing or suctioning, which transiently raise ICP, or due to head-of-bed manipulation. Theoretically, clamping the EVD during these events can temper this risk.

Is there an increased risk of cerebrospinal fluid infection with continuous vs. intermittent drainage?

In addition to fears of overdrainage and potential ventricular collapse, opponents of continuous CSF drainage cite the increased infection rates with an open EVD. Ventriculitis remains a valid concern and will be subsequently discussed.

What is the role of continuous cerebrospinal fluid drainage in subarachnoid hemorrhage?

Vasospasm, delayed cerebral ischemia, hydrocephalus, and cerebral edema are complications of SAH. Although the pathogenesis of vasospasm is still unclear, one common theory associates the breakdown of blood products in the CSF with the formation of arterial vasospasm, suggesting that these blood products serve as spasmogens. Furthermore, the timeline of vasospasm appears to correlate with the stages of the breakdown of red blood cells (RBCs) while the resolution of vasospasm also appears to correlate with the clearing of blood from the CSF. It has therefore been postulated that continuous CSF drainage reduces the amount of blood products circulating in the CSF and may reduce the incidence of vasospasm compared to intermittent CSF drainage (22). In the past 5 years, one randomized controlled trial has addressed this hypothesis. Olson et al randomized patients within 72 hours of admission to either continuous CSF drainage with intermittent ICP monitoring or continuous ICP monitoring with intermittent drainage (23). An interim analysis was performed after

60 patients had been enrolled, and the study was halted due to a substantially higher incidence of complications in the continuous drainage group compared to the intermittent group. The most frequent complication was a nonpatent EVD that required frequent flushing or replacing (44.1% of patients in the continuous drainage group). The rate of ventriculitis was higher in the continuous CSF drainage group, at 17.6% compared to 3.8% in the intermittent group. This finding was not statistically significant, but a trend toward significance was present. Assessing the rate of vasospasm was the study's primary outcome, and though the trial ended early a trend toward significance favored the continuous CSF drainage group. Of the open-EVD group, 64.7% experienced vasospasm by any method (transcranial Doppler [TCD], angiogram, computed tomographic angiography [CTA]), compared to 80.8% of the ICP-monitor group. This study did not assess the rate of clinically significant symptomatic vasospasm or delayed cerebral ischemia between the two groups. However, assuming that patients taken for an angiogram warranted this more invasive intervention, 20.6% of patients in the open-EVD group were found to have vasospasm present via angiogram, compared to 34.6% in the ICP-monitor group. The total CSF output was approximately equal in both groups. This study's sample size of 60 patients was too small to fully explore the hypothesis regarding the effect of continuous drainage on vasospasm, but this was likely due to the trial halting prematurely. Also, the groups were unequal in their distribution, with 26 patients in the intermittent drainage group compared to 34 patients in the continuous group. Two prospective observational studies published prior to this trial seem to corroborate the findings of more EVD-related complications with continuous drainage. They found a nonsignificant but perhaps clinically meaningful discovery of increased ventriculitis (24). These findings fuel the need for further studies not only to assess the effect of these two CSF drainage methods on the incidence of vasospasm in SAH but also to investigate the complication rate.

What role does continuous cerebrospinal fluid drainage play in traumatic brain injury?

As in SAH, no class I evidence exists regarding the role of continuous vs. intermittent CSF drainage in TBI patients, and a randomized controlled trial has not been performed as of this publication. As previously stated, a study in a pediatric population determined that continuous drainage resulted in decreased biomarkers of neuronal injury and an improved mean ICP (18). Another retrospective study conducted in an adult population demonstrated a greater mean ICP in patients receiving intermittent drainage compared to continuous CSF drainage. However, there was no statistical difference in the incidence of CSF infection between the two groups (25), as compared to the SAH study (23). Another observational study found the rate of ventriculitis in TBI patients to be 8.3% with continuous CSF drainage (26). No statistical difference was noted in either survival or the GCS scale at 6 months. These data reinforce the need for a randomized controlled trial to fully assess the impact of these two drainage strategies in TBI.

THE ROLE OF INTRACRANIAL PRESSURE MONITORING IN ACUTE LIVER FAILURE

CASE STUDY *A 32-year-old male admitted to the ICU after an acetaminophen overdose with acute liver failure (ALF) awaiting liver transplantation becomes unarousable and is intubated. A CT scan of the brain compared to his CT scan on presentation reveals sulcal effacement and open but compressed ventricles (Figure 3.1). He is determined to have grade IV encephalopathy, and his ammonia level is 175 µmol/L. The neurological intensive care team is consulted due to concerns of intracranial hypertension.*

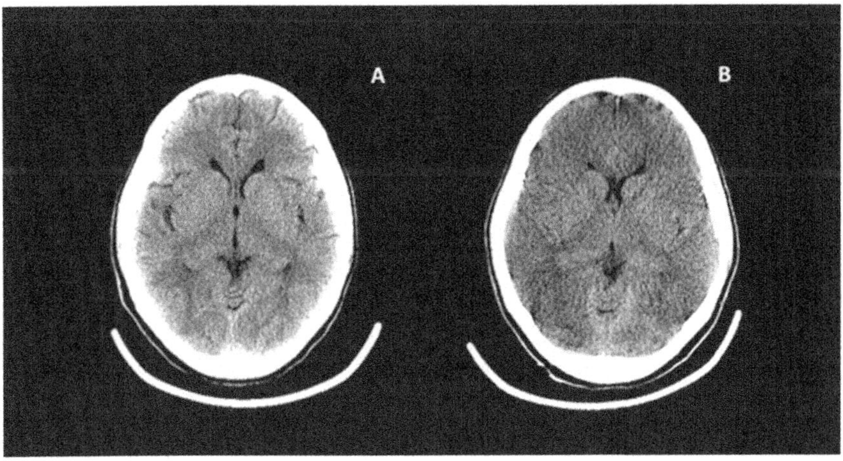

FIGURE 3.1 (A) CT brain without contrast. No evidence of cerebral edema. (B) CT showing loss of differentiation of the gray-white junction and loss of sulci with diffuse cerebral edema.

What is the mechanism of cerebral edema in acute liver failure?

The mechanism remains unclear but is thought to be due to concomitant factors. Ammonia appears to play a significant role, and a close relationship exists between the level of serum ammonia and the degree of clinically observed encephalopathy. Astrocytes are the cells most susceptible to the sudden increase in arterial ammonia levels present in ALF. Astrocytes contain the enzyme glutamine synthetase, which is involved in the conversion of ammonia to glutamine. This increase in intracellular glutamine results in increased intracellular osmolarity, drawing water into the astrocyte and thereby increasing ICP. Ammonia is also directly neurotoxic and negatively affects neurotransmitters, causes impaired energy metabolism, and disrupts cerebral blood flow autoregulation (27). A serum ammonia level of 150 to 200 µmol/L is closely correlated with a higher probability of elevated ICP (28). Intracranial hypertension was previously the leading cause of mortality in patients with ALF; however, the prevalence of intracranial hypertension in this population has decreased with the advent of emergency liver transplantation and aggressive medical management (29). The most common cause of ALF in North America is acetaminophen toxicity (28). Intracranial hypertension and brain edema tend to develop more often in younger patients and appear to be more prevalent in females compared to males (29,30).

Are there guidelines or possible indications for intracranial pressure monitoring in the setting of acute liver failure?

The U.S. Acute Liver Failure Study Group recommends ICP monitoring in patients with West Haven Criteria grade III or grade IV hepatic encephalopathy (Table 3.2). It is estimated that 25% to 35% of patients with grade III encephalopathy and 65% to 75% of patients with grade IV encephalopathy develop intracranial hypertension (31). A large retrospective review performed in the United Kingdom found that 41.8% of patients admitted to an ICU specializing in liver failure between 1973 and 2008 had signs consistent with intracranial hypertension. Patients with intracranial hypertension had a survival rate of 26.4%, compared to 52.5% in those without intracranial hypertension (29). However, despite these recommendations there remains wide discord from center to center in the monitoring of patients with ALF. Physicians remain reluctant to place monitors in these patients because of an increased procedural hemorrhagic risk due to the coagulopathic state of ALF. One study estimated that the probability of receiving ICP monitoring in patients with grade IV

TABLE 3.2 West Haven criteria grades of hepatic encephalopathy

Grade	Characteristic/Symptoms
I	Trivial lack of awareness Euphoria or anxiety Shortened attention span Impaired performance of addition or subtraction
II	Lethargy or apathy Minimal disorientation for time or place Subtle personality change Inappropriate behavior
III	Somnolence to semistupor, but responsive to verbal stimuli Confusion Gross disorientation
IV	Coma (unresponsive to verbal or noxious stimuli)

hepatic encephalopathy was between 0% and 85% depending on the center (30). Proponents of ICP monitoring state that ICP monitors allow for the accurate calculation of cerebral perfusion pressure, especially in the setting of cerebrovascular dysregulation, common in liver failure. They believe that monitoring assists in assessing the response to ICP-lowering treatments while providing valuable information that can help determine the eligibility for liver transplantation. Proponents also assert that the risk of catastrophic brain hemorrhage is lower compared to the risk of mortality and morbidity from ALF itself.

CASE STUDY *The patient meets the criteria for an emergency liver transplantation, and the decision is made to proceed. The head of the bed is raised to 30 degrees and propofol is started. He is given mannitol 1.5 g/kg, and neurosurgery is consulted for an ICP monitor placement prior to his being taken to the operating room. However, he is thrombocytopenic, with a platelet count of 89,000/mcL and an international normalized ratio (INR) of 4.6 and prolonged prothrombin time.*

What international normalized ratio value and platelet value should be targeted prior to placing an intracranial pressure monitor in patients with acute liver failure?

Neurosurgeons typically aim for an INR of less than 1.6 and a platelet count greater than 100,000/mcL prior to ICP monitor placement to minimize bleeding risk. The U.S. Acute Liver Failure Study Group's study assessing complications of ICP monitoring in ALF patients found a low incidence of intracerebral hemorrhage, with four out of 56 patients (7%) who received ICP monitors of any type experiencing hemorrhagic complications. This study did not assess the possible correlation, if any, between the type of monitor placed and the complication rate. This finding corroborated a prior study that found 10% of patients experienced some degree of intracerebral hemorrhage after ICP monitor placement (32). It should be noted, however, that three of the four patients who had intracerebral hemorrhage later died. The etiology of death is not explicitly stated in the paper. It is unclear if these deaths were secondary to the intracerebral hemorrhage itself or if these patients had a higher risk of bleeding due to the increased severity of their liver failure, which ultimately resulted in their deaths.

Which type of monitor will reduce the risk of hemorrhage?

Most physicians believe there is a reduced risk of intracranial hemorrhage with the placement of a bolt, a type of monitor that measures only ICP. Bolts are inserted with a fiber-optic transducer. EVDs are rarely, if ever, used in this patient population secondary to hemorrhagic concerns. Furthermore, there is debate on whether the ICP monitor should be placed in the epidural or subdural space or if an intraparenchymal device can be used. In one retrospective study, 58 patients with ALF had ICP monitors placed. Most patients had subdural transducers placed (63.8%), followed by intraparenchymal devices (20.7%) and epidural transducers (15.5%). No intraventricular catheter use was reported. Six of these 58 patients (10%) had intracranial hemorrhages; three patients had symptomatic intracerebral hemorrhage (ICH). The highest incidence of ICH was observed in patients who had subdural catheters (four out of six patients), and one incidence of ICH occurred in each of the epidural and intraparenchymal groups. Three patients who received ICP monitoring died, two due to brain edema and one due to refractory hypotension. No death was attributed to the placement of an ICP monitor (33). These results are similar to those from an older study that found the highest hemorrhagic complication rate with subdural monitors. No use of intraventricular catheters was reported (34). The final decision of what type of monitor to place often ultimately depends on the neurosurgeon and institutional familiarity, but it appears as though subdural fiber-optic placement carries the highest bleeding risk.

What can be done to correct the coagulopathy caused by acute liver failure?

Factors II, V, VII, IX, X, and XII are made in the liver. In ALF there is loss of both procoagulant and anticoagulant factors; the extent of liver damage correlates with the extent of coagulopathy. As both proclotting and anticlotting factors are lost, there remains a degree of homeostasis, and spontaneous bleeding is uncommon (28). However, during invasive procedures the risk of bleeding is elevated. The administration of vitamin K, fresh frozen plasma (FFP), and platelets is used to improve the coagulopathic state encountered in ALF prior to ICP monitor placement.

What is recombinant activated factor VII, and can it be used to correct this coagulopathy?

Initially approved for use in hemophiliacs, recombinant activated factor VII (rFVIIa) has been increasingly used off-label to aid in hemostasis and the emergent correction of coagulopathies. rFVIIa activates the coagulation cascade's extrinsic pathway, leading to thrombin and fibrin production. One recent meta-analysis evaluated the use of rFVIIa in patients with liver failure undergoing invasive procedures, with two retrospective cohort studies specifically examining the placement of ICP monitors in patients with fulminant hepatic failure (35). In one study, 11 consecutive coagulopathic patients having an average INR of 3.0 had intraparenchymal ICP monitors placed after receiving rFVIIa via an intravenous bolus, with an average dose of 36.7 mcg/kg. Patients also received FFP, packed RBCs, and platelets as needed. An ICP monitor was placed within 15 minutes to 2 hours of administering rFVIIa without rechecking coagulation studies due to the 2-hour half-life of rFVIIa and the fear of delaying intervention in patients with intracranial hypertension (31). No procedural-related complications (namely, hemorrhage) occurred in this small cohort of patients, but further prospective studies with a larger sample size have yet to be performed.

What dose of recombinant activated factor VII should be given prior to placing an intracranial pressure monitor?

The length of coagulation correction depends on the dose of rFVIIa—the higher the dose, the longer the length of coagulation correction. There is no standard dose of rFVIIa, but it is suggested that a dose of 20 to 40 mcg/kg seems to be optimal for invasive procedures (35). A previous study demonstrated that a dose of rFVIIa of 40 mcg/kg reduced INR to less than 1.6. This dose allowed ICP monitors to be placed in seven patients with fulminant hepatic failure, correcting their coagulopathic state within 30 minutes of administration. However, eight other patients were given FFP alone, and only three of these had coagulopathic states corrected to a level that facilitated ICP monitor placement (36).

What should be considered prior to administering recombinant activated factor VII?

rFVIIa administration leads to an increased risk of arterial thromboembolic events. The risk increases with higher medication dosages. A recently published Cochrane review evaluating the effectiveness and safety of rFVIIa cautioned against its off-label use due to arterial thrombosis, resulting in events such as myocardial infarction, pulmonary embolism, hepatic artery thrombosis, or stroke (37). Another meta-analysis found a rate of 5.5% of arterial thromboembolic events compared to placebo (3.2%), with no increase in the rate of venous thromboembolic events (38). In addition to this legitimate risk, rFVIIa is expensive and costs $1,000 to $1,500 per milligram on average. The cost-benefit ratio should be considered prior to administration (35). For these reasons, the lowest possible dose to achieve reversal of the patient's coagulopathic state should be administered, and only after carefully discussing it with the team and the patient or patient's proxy and performing a detailed risk-benefit analysis.

Does intracranial pressure monitoring improve outcomes in patients with acute liver failure?

Much debate in general has taken place over the role of ICP monitoring in many conditions and disease states. In a large cohort of patients with ALF who received ICP monitoring, it did not appear to improve mortality in acetaminophen-induced ALF and was actually associated with worse outcomes in non–acetaminophen-induced ALF (32). Sicker patients with multiorgan failure and overt intracranial hypertension and cerebral edema, however, are more likely to have ICP monitors placed, and this may have influenced this finding. Future prospective studies are needed to answer this question definitively.

INTRACRANIAL PRESSURE MONITORING AFTER CARDIAC ARREST

Very little data are available in vivo to determine the reversibility of brain dysfunction after cardiac arrest. Acute ischemia from hypoperfusion during arrest results in cerebral edema, causing elevations in ICP and acute changes in brain tissue energy metabolites, which can be measured with cerebral microdialysis methods. Human data show acute rises in extracellular lactate to pyruvate ratios as well as elevated glycerol levels after cardiac arrest (39,40). This suggests a failure of brain energy metabolism and cell membrane breakdown. Additionally, ICP in these two case series was not elevated during the time of monitoring.

Can it be done safely?

Although intracranial monitoring of brain pressure and physiology is not routinely done after cardiac arrest, some data are available in the literature. A small case series from Sweden describes four patients treated with therapeutic hypothermia and intracranial monitoring after cardiac arrest. ICP was monitored along with cerebral microdialysis for 35 to 40 hours post–cardiac arrest. All four patients achieved a good neurological outcome, with recovery of baseline or almost baseline cognitive and motor function (40).

Is it useful?

Experimental models show some evidence that under extremely controlled circumstances of cardiac arrest under deep hypothermia, reperfusion techniques can mitigate the rise of ICP and the derangements of cellular metabolism seen with microdialysis. Histology also confirms a decrease in apoptotic cells with these techniques (41). Thus, ICP monitoring and microdialysis may be able to detect improvement in brain tissue chemistry and edema after cardiac arrest. This could potentially lead to improved clinical outcome. In humans we know that about a quarter of patients will have elevated ICP after cardiac arrest and that this is a poor prognostic sign (42). Interestingly, a more recent case series from Sweden (41) demonstrated significant derangements in brain energy metabolites during and after cardiac arrest. All four patients had significant and persistent elevations in extracellular glycerol. This represents membrane breakdown and tissue destruction and was seen in all patients despite clinical improvement. Additionally, all patients had brain tissue microdialysis showing an elevation in the lactate to pyruvate ratio. This is typically associated with tissue ischemia and is understandably seen during and after cardiac arrest. However, although three of the four patients showed initial elevations in the lactate to pyruvate ratio not all of them normalized, and one patient showed a secondary rise in the lactate to pyruvate ratio that was considerable with rewarming. Unfortunately, none of these patterns tended to correlate with any clinical change or outcome measure. Perhaps one explanation is that the sample of tissue monitored with the microdialysis probe is quite small and may not represent global changes in tissue chemistry. It is also possible that these alterations in tissue chemistry are signatures of the initial ischemic injury suffered during the arrest and do not represent a modifiable target. A more recent case series of cerebral microdialysis included two patients with cardiac arrest and demonstrated an association between mortality and a reduced brain serum glucose ratio (43). Brain tissue hypoglycemia and inadequate substrate for adenosine triphosphate (ATP) production to support neuronal metabolism may explain this. Although this may be a modifiable target, the available data cannot demonstrate reversibility. Concomitantly, when Nordmark et al measured ICP after cardiac arrest it did not rise in any of the patients studied (40,44). This may be explained by the fact that all of these patients had a good outcome. We do know that patients who do poorly are more likely to have cerebral edema and therefore are expected to have an elevated ICP. This, however, does not necessarily mean that treating their ICP will change the poor outcome. Interestingly, in a series of eight comatose patients post–cardiac arrest who were treated with a therapeutic hypothermia protocol and monitored with ICP monitoring, cerebral microdialysis, and near-infrared spectroscopy (NIRS), none had elevated ICP despite the induction of hypercapnia during the study protocol (44). This concept was also demonstrated in a small case series of patients who had ICP monitoring after malignant cerebral infarction (45). In this series the authors showed that ICP monitors can be placed in patients who have had decompressive craniectomies for the treatment of malignant anterior circulation ischemic strokes. Many patients developed elevations in the ICP for varying amounts of time. Most of these episodes responded well to traditional measures used to lower ICP (CSF drainage, osmotics, mild hyperventilation, and sedation). However, these episodes and their treatment had no effect on the ultimate clinical outcome. The outcome was determined, as expected, by the patient's age and National Institutes of Health stroke scale (NIHSS).

It is possible that brain injury sustained after cardiac arrest is modifiable. A recent meta-analysis of studies examining respiratory parameters after cardiac arrest found normoxia to be associated with a decrease in mortality when compared with hypoxia and hyperoxia in an adult population. Oxygenation and ventilation have significant effects on brain perfusion and energy metabolism after injury, and these findings may suggest an opportunity to optimize modifiable targets (46). Unfortunately, we do not have convincing evidence that intracranial monitoring post–cardiac arrest provides such a modifiable target.

CASE STUDY *A 24-year-old male single-person motorcycle accident, unhelmeted, presents to the emergency room with a GCS score of 5; 4 mm, round, and briskly reactive pupils; and evidence of bifrontal contusions in the head CT. Alcohol level: 0.384.*

In intoxicated patients with traumatic brain injuries, how long is it reasonable to wait before placing an intracranial monitor?

Alcohol intoxication has been reported in up to 50% of patients admitted after TBI (47,48). In the United States, alcohol misuse has been identified as the leading risk factor for serious injury (48). In 2010 Shahin et al found, in a retrospective study, that admission GCS scores in intoxicated patients often improved by two points on day one after admission. Intoxication was defined as a blood alcohol concentration (BAC) greater than 0.08%. A BAC of 0.08% is the legal upper limit for driving in most of the United States because some motor and cognitive impairment is present at this level (47,49). The GCS improvement was associated with an improvement from severe (GCS: 3–8) to moderate (GCS: 9–12) TBI. This is frequently the determining factor for ICP monitor placement. Also, lower GCS scores on admission led to more significant improvements in best GCS scores on day one after admission. The amount of improvement in the GCS score from admission to the best score on day one was also directly related to BAC. Some protocols include closely monitoring intoxicated patients with TBI for an interval of 6 hours before assigning the admission GCS score (47).

In 2010 Hadjizacharia et al (48) reported retrospective data from a level I trauma center. Data assessing outcome in trauma patients after alcohol exposure were collected between 2002 and 2005. They identified 386 patients with positive alcohol screening (AP) and matched each with a single patient with negative alcohol screening (AN) based on demographic characteristics. Specifically, age, gender, mechanism of injury (blunt vs. penetrating), injury severity score (ISS), head abbreviated injury score (AIS), chest AIS, abdominal AIS, and extremities AIS were the matched variables. Characteristic differences between groups were not significant, except that the AN group had a greater incidence of hemopneumothorax. Overall mortality as well as the incidence of hypotension (systolic BP less than 90 mmHg) was significantly increased in the AP group, and GCS scores were less than 8 upon admission. In-house cardiac arrest incidence was also higher in the AP group, which may suggest an interaction between alcohol ingestion and cardiovascular instability.

We know that alcohol intoxication depresses the GCS score, and we know that patients with alcohol intoxication can also have severe injuries (47,48). Rundhaug et al (50) recommend considering CT findings on admission when making a final decision on how long to wait to determine injury severity. In this cohort study, they used Rotterdam CT scores (see Table 3.3) on admission to stratify patients according to injury severity and correlate this to BAC levels and GCS scores during the hospitalization period. They compared patients with Rotterdam scores of 1 to 3 (group 1) vs. 4 to 6 (group 2) and concluded that BAC seemed to have more effect on GCS scores in patients in group 1 upon admission. Group 2 included the patients with CT findings suggesting intracranial hypertension. They concluded that even though BAC affects global GCS scores, the management of severe brain injuries should not be delayed due to alcohol's central nervous system (CNS)–depressing effect in patients with a higher Rotterdam score. Although one must always consider the possibility of a severe brain injury due to axonal shearing in patients with a low Rotterdam CT score, the authors suggest that this approach can be cautiously considered when examining intoxicated patients.

TABLE 3.3 Rotterdam CT score (0 to 6)[10]

CT Findings	Score
Basal Cisterns	
Normal	0
Compressed	1
Absent	2
Midline Shift	
No shift or <5mm	0
Shift >5mm	1
Epidural Mass Lesion	
Present	0
Absent	1
Intraventricular Blood (IVH) or Subarachnoid Hemorrhage (SAH)	
Absent	0
Present	1

The synergism between alcohol, CNS-depressing effects, and acute brain injury influencing GCS scores during the first hours after injury should be considered when evaluating this population. A balance between careful observation and aggressive early treatment should be sought when taking into consideration the trauma mechanism and imaging findings in patients with alcohol intoxication and severe TBI (50).

References

1. Chesnut RM, Temkin N, Carney N, et al. A trial of intracranial pressure monitoring in traumatic brain injury. *New Engl J Med.* 2012;367(26):2471–2481.

2. Carney N, Lujan S, Dikmen S, et al. Intracranial pressure monitoring in severe traumatic brain injury in Latin America: process and methods for a multi-center randomized controlled trial. *J Neurotrauma.* 2012;29:2022–2029.

3. Bratton S, Bullock MR, Carney N, et al. Guidelines for management of severe TBI. *J Neurotrauma.* 2007;24:S1–106.

4. O'Phelan KH, Park D, Efird JT, et al. Patterns of increased intracranial pressure after traumatic brain injury. *Neurocrit Care.* 2009;10(3):280–286.

5. Chestnut RM. A conceptual approach to managing severe traumatic brain injury in a time of uncertainty. *Ann N Y Acad Sci.* 2014;16:1–9.

6. Chestnut RM. Intracranial pressure monitoring: headstone or a new head start. The BEST TRIP trial in perspective. *Intensive Care Med.* 2013;39(4):771–774.

7. Le Roux P. Intracranial pressure after the BEST TRIP trial: a call for more monitoring. *Curr Opin Crit Care.* 2014;20(2):141–147.

8. Murillo-Cabezas F, Godoy DA. [Intracranial pressure monitoring in severe traumatic brain injury: A different perspective of the BestTrip trial] [article in Spanish]. *Medicina Intensiva.* 2014;38(4):237–239.

9. Jennett B J, Teasdale G, Galbaith S, et al. Severe head injuries in three countries. *J Neurol Neurosurg Psychiatry.* 1977;40:290–298.

10. Marshall LF, Becker DP, Bowers SA, et al. The National Traumatic Coma Data Bank. *J Neurosurg.* 1983;59:276–284.

11. Rosner MJ, Becker DP. Origin and evolution of plateau waves. *J Neurosurg.* 1984;60: 312–324.

12. Lundberg N. Continuous recording and control of ventricular fluid pressure in neurosurgical practice. *Acta Psychiatr Scand.* 1960;36(149):1–193.

13. Allen BB, Chiu Y, Gerber LM, et al. Age specific cerebral perfusion pressure thresholds and survival in children and adolescents with severe traumatic brain injury. *Pediatr Crit Care Med.* 2014;15:62–70.

14. Kiening KL, Schoening W, Unterberg AW, et al. Assessment of the relationship between age and continuous intracranial compliance. *Acta Neurochir Suppl.* 2005;95:293–297.

15. Czosnyka M, Smielewski P, Kirkpatrick P, et al. *Neurosurg.* 1997;41(1):11–19.

16. Lazaridis C, DeSantis SM, Smeilewski P, et al. Patient-specific thresholds of intracranial pressure in severe traumatic brain injury. *J Neurosurgery.* 2014;120:893–900.

17. Vender J, Waller J, Dhandapani K, et al. An evaluation and comparison of intraventricular, intraparenchymal, and fluid-coupled techniques for intracranial pressure monitoring in patients with severe traumatic brain injury. *J Clin Monit Comput.* 2011;25(4):231–236.

18. Shore PM, Thomas NJ, Clark RS, et al. Continuous versus intermittent cerebrospinal fluid drainage after severe traumatic brain injury in children: effect on biochemical markers. *J Neurotrauma*. 2004;21:1113–1122.

19. Exo J, Kochanek PM, Adelson PD, et al. Intracranial pressure-monitoring systems in children with traumatic brain injury: combining therapeutic and diagnostic tools. *Pediatr Crit Care Med*. 2011;12:560–565.

20. Wolfla CE, Luerssen TG, Bowman RM, et al. Brain tissue pressure gradients created by expanding frontal epidural mass lesion. *J Neurosurg*. 1996;84:642–647.

21. *Integra Design Verification Report for Camino Flex Ventricular Catheter*. 49–51.

22. Kim G, Amato A, James M, et al. Continuous and intermittent CSF diversion after subarachnoid hemorrhage: a pilot study. *Neurocrit Care*. 2011;14:68–72.

23. Olson DM, Zomorodi M, Britz GW, et al. Continuous cerebral spinal fluid drainage associated with complications in patients admitted with subarachnoid hemorrhage: clinical article. *J Neurosurg*. 2013;119:974–980.

24. Amato A, Britz GW, James ML, et al. An observational pilot study of CSF diversion in subarachnoid haemorrhage. *Nurs Crit Care*. 2011;16:252–260.

25. Nwachuku EL, Puccio AM, Fetzick A, et al. Intermittent versus continuous cerebrospinal fluid drainage management in adult severe traumatic brain injury: assessment of intracranial pressure burden. *Neurocrit Care*. 2014;20:49–53.

26. Andrade AF, Paiva WS, Amorim, RL, et al. Continuous ventricular cerebrospinal fluid drainage with intracranial pressure monitoring for management of posttraumatic diffuse brain swelling. *Arq Neuropsiquiatr*. 2011;69:79–84.

27. Seyan AS, Hughes RD, Shawcross DL. Changing face of hepatic encephalopathy: role of inflammation and oxidative stress. *World J Gastroenterol*. 2010;16:3347–3357.

28. Bernal W, Wendon J. Acute liver failure. *N Engl J Med*. 2013;369:2525–2534.

29. Bernal W, Hyyrylainen A, Gera A, et al. Lessons from look-back in acute liver failure? a single centre experience of 3300 patients. *J Hepatol*. 2013;59:74–80.

30. Vaquero J, Fontana RJ, Larson AM, et al. Complications and use of intracranial pressure monitoring in patients with acute liver failure and severe encephalopathy. *Liver Transpl*. 2005;11:1581–1589.

31. Shami VM, Caldwell SH, Hespenheide EE, et al. Recombinant activated factor VII for coagulopathy in fulminant hepatic failure compared with conventional therapy. *Liver Transpl*. 2003;9:138–143.

32. Karvellas CJ, Fix OK, Battenhouse H, et al. Outcomes and complications of intracranial pressure monitoring in acute liver failure: a retrospective cohort study. *Crit Care Med*. 2014;42:1157–1167.

33. Vaquero J, Fontana RJ, Larson AM, et al. Complications and use of intracranial pressure monitoring in patients with acute liver failure and severe encephalopathy. *Liver Transpl*. 2005;11:1581–1589.

34. Blei A, Olafsson S, Webster S, et al. Complications of intracranial pressure monitoring in fulminant hepatic failure. *Lancet*. 1993;341:157–158.

35. Krisl JC, Meadows HE, Greenberg CS, et al. Clinical usefulness of recombinant activated factor VII in patients with liver failure undergoing invasive procedures. *Ann Pharmacother*. 2011;45:1433–1438.

36. Le TV, Rumbak MJ, Liu SS, et al. Insertion of intracranial pressure monitors in fulminant hepatic failure patients: early experience using recombinant factor VII. *Neurosurgery*. 2010;66:455,8;(discussion):458.

37. Simpson E, Lin Y, Stanworth S, et al. Recombinant factor VIIa for the prevention and treatment of bleeding in patients without haemophilia. In: *Cochrane Database of Systematic Reviews*. 2012(3): CD005011. doi: 10.1002/14651858.CD005011.pub4.

38. Levi M, Levy JH, Andersen HF, et al. Safety of recombinant activated factor VII in randomized clinical trials. *N Engl J Med*. 2010;363:1791–1800.

39. Bauer R, Gabl M, Obwegeser A, et al. Neurochemical monitoring using intracerebral microdialysis during cardiac resuscitation. *Intensive Care Med*. 2004;30:159–161.

40. Nordmark J, Rubertsson S, Mortberg E, et al. Intracerebral monitoring in comatose patients treated with hypothermia after cardiac arrest. *Acta Anesthesiol Scand*. 2009;53:289–298.

41. Liang M, Tang Z, Chen G, et al. Is selective antegrade cerebral perfusion superior to retrograde cerebral perfusion for brain protection during deep hypothermic cardiac arrest? metabolic evidence from microdialysis. *Crit Care Med*. 2014;42:e319–e328.

42. Gueugniaud PY, Garcia-Darennes F, Gaussorgues P, et al. Prognostic significance of early intracranial and cerebral perfusion pressures in post cardiac arrest anoxic coma. *Intensive Care Med*. 1991;17(7):392–398.

43. Kurtz P, Claassen, Schmidt JM, et al. Reduced brain/serum glucose ratios predict cerebral metabolic distress and mortality after severe brain injury. *Neurocrit Care*. 2013;19: 311–319.

44. Pynnonen L, Falkenbach P, Kamarainen A, et al. Therapeutic hypothermia after cardiac arrest—cerebral perfusion and metabolism during upper and lower threshold normocapnia. *Resuscitation*. 2011;82:1174–1179.

45. Paldor I, Rosenthal G, Cohen JE, et al. Intracranial pressure monitoring following decompressive hemicraniectomy for malignant cerebral infarction. *J Clin Neurosci*. 2015;22: 79–82.

46. Suthersan Y, Vargas M, Brunetti I, et al. Ventilatory targets after cardiac arrest. *Minerva Anestesiol*. 2015;81:39–51.

47. Shahin H, Gopinath SP, Robertson CS. Influence of alcohol on early Glasgow Coma Scale in head-injured patients. *J Neurotrauma*. 2010;69(5):1176–1181.

48. Hadjizacharia P, O'Keeffe T, Plurad DS, et al. Alcohol exposure and outcomes in trauma patients. *Eur J Trauma Emerg Surg*. 2011;37(2):169–175.

49. Hsieh CH, Su LT, Wang YC, et al. Does alcohol intoxication protect patients with severe injury and reduce hospital mortality? The association of alcohol consumption with the severity of injury and survival in trauma patients. *American Surgeon*. 2013;(79)12:1289–1294.

50. Rundhaug NP, Moen KG, Skandsen T, et al. Moderate and severe traumatic brain injury: effect of blood alcohol concentration on Glasgow Coma Scale score and relation to computed tomography findings. *J Neurosurgery*. 2015;122(1):211–218.

Cerebral Herniation Syndromes 4

Scott A. Marshall
Adam M. Willis

INTRODUCTION

The clinical consequences of compartmentalized intracranial pressure (ICP) may yield predictable exam findings that can localize the causal intracranial space-occupying lesions. Particular neurologic structures suffering injury from this phenomenon are referred to as *cerebral herniation syndromes*. Inherent to this topic is both the cause and effect; ie, typically with elevations in intracerebral pressure, the resulting displacement of neuronal structures causes the subsequent syndrome of clinical manifestations. Because of the predictable clinical patterns found in herniation syndromes, along with the potential for intervention (and the devastating consequences if not treated promptly), common and uncommon types of cerebral herniation syndromes encountered clinically and radiographically in the neurocritical care environment should be understood. Traumatic brain injury (TBI) is likely the most common clinical condition in which herniation syndromes play out in the neurosciences critical care unit (NCCU), although essentially any condition that results in a space-occupying lesion and the elevation of ICP can produce a cerebral herniation syndrome.

When the intracranial vault is kept intact, the components therein exist in a variable ratio but typically exist in a state of mechanical equilibrium. If the volume of one component of the contents of the cranium increases or decreases, the remaining intracranial components must also decrease or increase to maintain a fixed total volume. The normal intracranial components include brain tissue, cerebrospinal fluid (CSF), and blood (both venous and arterial components).

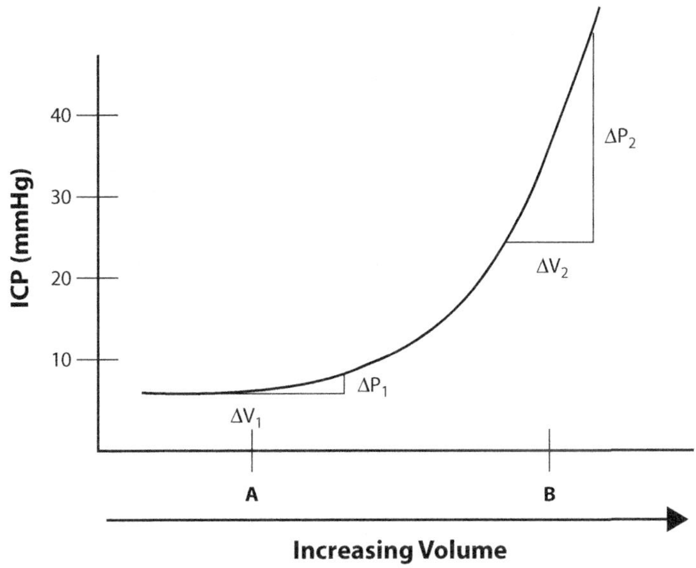

FIGURE 4.1 Intracranial compliance curve showing how small changes in volume result in small changes in pressure as compensation is maintained. As a critical volume is reached, small changes in volume result in large changes in pressure. *Note:* ICP, intracranial pressure.

In pathologic states, cerebral edema (brain), hydrocephalus or intraventricular blood (CSF), or epidural and subdural hematomas (SDHs) force compensatory volume changes from the surrounding brain, CSF, and intravascular blood. This relationship has perhaps been most memorably described by Monro and Kellie and is commonly taught using their eponymous doctrine (1,2), whereby slowly progressing increases or decreases in the volume of one intracranial component may not alter the ICP because compensatory mechanisms maintain optimal pressures. However, rapid changes may not allow these compensatory mechanisms to occur, thereby altering the dynamics of blood and CSF flow as well as producing dramatic increases in pressure. Additionally, because of the nonlinear compliance curve of intracranial contents as volumes increase, the resultant change in pressure from a change in volume monotonically increases. Thus, moderate changes in volume result in small differences in ICP; however, as volumes continue to grow, subsequently smaller increases in intracranial volume result in larger relative changes in ICP (Figure 4.1).

In the NCCU setting, these patients often have acute space-occupying lesions, such as an acute SDH, or a chronic lesion, such as a brain tumor, which has progressed over time to a point where compensatory mechanisms can no longer effectively maintain equilibrium. In this situation ICP rises and, if left unchecked, can result in the clinical and radiographic presentation of a cerebral herniation syndrome.

THE EXAMINATION OF NEUROLOGICALLY INJURED PATIENTS

The clinical examination of a patient with a suspected acquired brain injury, whether from trauma, brain tumor, idiopathic hemorrhage, or metabolic derangements, has both prognostic and management implications. The question, "When did this subtle pupil asymmetry occur?" or more commonly, "Is this patient still localizing or is this now a withdrawal response?" can unfortunately arise. Without careful, methodical, and frequent patient examinations, our most sensitive indicator of neurologic compromise in the NCCU is lost, and the patient is more often whisked off to the scanner where perhaps a radiographic anatomic change is found. In the setting of trauma, Advanced Trauma Life Support (ATLS) is a primary resource for providers who treat brain injuries This training emphasizes the careful and early documentation of a neurologic examination in all patients so that changes that occur in subsequent examinations can be recognized as such and acted upon swiftly (3). After ensuring that the patient's airway, breathing, and circulation are cared for, ATLS focuses next on a rapid initial neurological evaluation, especially to determine the patient's Glasgow Coma Scale (GCS) score (3,4). The GCS score is important for triage and is a quantifiable measure of impairment that can help decide early management sequences. This initial exam also helps prognosticate the outcome of moderate and severe TBI and penetrating TBI (5,6). The GCS should ideally be described not in an aggregate score but broken down into its components, particularly to qualify motor function (4). Assessment of the patient's pupils, extraocular muscles, and motor examination (desirably in a more granular and specific evaluation of motor function than simply an "M" score) are probably the most vital components of the initial neurologic exam. Along with changes in the patient's vital signs and mental status, many, if not all, of the cerebral herniation syndromes can be diagnosed from changes in these three areas of the neurologic examination.

THE CAUSES OF CEREBRAL HERNIATION

As discussed, cerebral herniation occurs due to changes in intracerebral pressure or compartmentalized pressure differences between regions of the brain.

These compartmentalized pressure gradients reach a yielding threshold whereby the normal anatomical configuration can no longer support such a gradient, and intracranial contents are displaced. This displacement often causes the disruption of neuroanatomic structures or the regional vascular supply (7). Because both focal low and high pressures can result in a pressure gradient, not all cerebral herniation occurs with gross elevations in pressure, as is the case with the infrequently encountered low pressure herniation, or paradoxical herniation syndrome, discussed later. In general, however, the cause of herniation is most often an end-state of unchecked or untenable elevations in ICP caused by a space-occupying lesion in the brain. This condition has many specific causes, including mass lesions, metabolic or osmotic derangements, and CSF or blood outflow obstruction. A brief discussion of some of these mechanisms follows; these processes are also reviewed in more detail in the first chapter of this book.

Space-Occupying or Mass Lesions

Clinicians managing the critical and emergency care of patients with intracranial mass effect typically encounter lesions such as SDH, epidural hematoma (EDH), intracerebral hemorrhage (ICH), intraventricular hemorrhage (IVH), and acute-on-chronic mass effect from a brain tumor as a cause of an impending cerebral herniation syndrome. As stated earlier, chronic or slow changes in the intracranial compliance relationship between volume and pressure are fairly well tolerated, up to a point. When this ability is exceeded, small increases in volume cause large increases in ICP (8). This relationship works in the opposite direction, also. Therapeutic interventions that remove small amounts of volume from the brain, such as CSF diversion or the evacuation of a hematoma, initiated when the brain in on the far right side of the compliance curve, may show quite drastic changes in measured ICP (Figure 4.1).

Patients frequently present to the NCCU with traumatic SDH. The projected incidence of SDH in the United States is expected to reach 60,000 cases annually by 2030, which would make it the most common cranial neurosurgical condition encountered in the future (9). These lesions can have acute or acute-on-chronic presentations and are easily diagnosed by routine imaging. Risk factors for the development of SDH include trauma, advanced age, and ongoing systemic anticoagulation (10). Depending on the presentation, SDH has a variable prognosis.

EDH can present in several locations but classically is described as occurring under a skull fracture that ruptures a meningeal artery. An EDH has the potential to increase in size rapidly and require urgent neurosurgical evaluation.

A torn dural vein likely causes the other mass lesions in the epidural space that are smaller and do not tend to increase in size when followed by serial CT scans. Nonetheless, a neurosurgeon should evaluate all EDHs due to the difficulty in predicting which will progress and may require urgent evacuation.

IVH can occur as an extension of ICH or be isolated. Blood products in the ventricular system can often result in an obstructive hydrocephalus and lead to a herniation syndrome. Additionally, vasogenic or extracellular edema from a malignant brain tumor can cause an acute-on-chronic mass effect, resulting in increased ICP and the potential to worsen intracranial compliance. Also, an acute worsening of the neurologic status of a patient with a known intracranial mass can occur when a patient hemorrhages into the mass, with resultant malignant cerebral edema (11).

Metabolic Derangements

Patients with systemic illness often have metabolic disorders that cause neurologic dysfunction. The hallmark of these disorders is often a presentation that is acute on chronic or subacute in onset. These patients present frequently in the NCCU, and neurocritical care physicians are often asked to render a consult opinion on the neurologic management of these patients when cared for in other intensive care units (ICUs). Common examples include liver and renal failure, glycemic derangements, hypercapnia, and hypoxia, among other causes.

Liver dysfunction and its progression to fulminant hepatic failure have consequences on intracranial compliance and can lead to herniation syndromes (12). The mechanism by which liver failure increases ICP is multifactorial, but several key mechanisms predominate. The cerebral edema that often accompanies liver failure is linked to ammonia accumulation, glutamate toxicity, and N-methyl-D-aspartate (NMDA) receptor activation. Specifically, ammonia concentrations unchecked by abnormal hepatic function cause metabolism to intracellular glutamine within the astrocyte that, in turn, raises intracellular osmotic pressure and results in fluid accumulation and edema within the astrocyte (12,13). In preclinical models, NMDA receptor stimulation also occurs in this setting, with resultant nitric oxide release and vasodilator effects in the brain (14). NMDA receptor antagonists may play a therapeutic role in this setting by reducing cerebral edema and interrupting herniation syndromes (15,16).

Likewise, renal insufficiency, either in combination with hepatic dysfunction or alone, may contribute to neurologic dysfunction, and secondary processes that follow renal failure can lead to poor intracranial compliance and contribute to herniation syndromes. A glomerular filtration rate less than or equal to

10% of normal, rather than absolute levels of either creatinine or urea, may be more associated with encephalopathy from renal causes, while the subsequent development of renal failure–induced electrolyte disorders, acidosis, seizures, and blood–brain barrier breakdown from proinflammatory mediators increases the risk of cerebral herniation (17). The treatment of renal failure can also be problematic, as shown in the reports of dialysis disequilibrium syndrome caused by rapid osmotic shifts and blood-brain gradients of intracellular urea from aggressive intermittent hemodialysis, but these cases have lessened since the increased use of continuous renal replacement therapy (CRRT) (18). Additionally, even in the setting of CRRT, death or neurologic injury from cerebral edema secondary to kidney failure can still occur, as the correction of underlying electrolyte, osmotic, and acid-base derangements can prove resistant to therapy (19).

Osmotic Derangements

Osmotic therapy likely represents the mainstay of treatment for an elevation in ICP, but comorbid processes may play a role in establishing electrolyte disorders that precipitate herniation syndromes. Pathological processes often result in osmotic gradients that are counterproductive for maintaining physiologic intracranial compliance. Derangements of serum sodium, commonly from the syndrome of inappropriate secretion of antidiuretic hormone (SIADH) and cerebral salt wasting (CSW), can alter brain tissue volume and exacerbate ICP gradients (20). Both CSW and SIADH have primary causes, including variations of acquired brain injury, the use of desmopressin for hemorrhage control, side effects from other medications, and malignancies (21,22). Paradoxically, hypernatremia can also be associated with a herniation syndrome in the correct clinical setting, as discussed later (23).

Cerebrospinal Fluid or Blood Flow Obstruction

An obstruction of normal outflow channels of either intracranial blood or CSF can cause a sudden increase in ICP that results in a herniation syndrome. In terms of CSF, cerebral herniation may result from obstructive hydrocephalus as a secondary consequence of other processes, eg, IVH or a tumor invading normal CSF outflow pathways (24). An increase in the volume of CSF within the intracranial compartment resulting from limitations of CSF outflow causes a caudal herniation of either supratentorial or infratentorial structures, or more rarely, increased drainage of CSF via extraventricular channels (ie, external ventricular drains) may cause herniation in a cephalad (upward) direction (25). The herniation syndromes associated with over- or underdrainage may present in an indolent manner and with more subtle clinical findings than typical cerebral herniation syndromes (26).

Similar to CSF outflow obstruction, the occlusion of a dural venous sinus due to thrombosis can result in increased ICP and cerebral herniation (27). The majority of intracranial blood is contained in venous, rather than arterial, capacitance vessels in the brain (28). The treatment of intracranial venous thrombus typically involves systemic or endovascular anticoagulation, but a delay in therapy can occur because ICH or SAH may be the initial finding in patients with occult dural venous sinus thrombosis (29,30). Although the Monro-Kellie doctrine would argue otherwise, isolated CSF shunting does not appear overly helpful in the management of patients with thrombosis of a venous sinus who cannot be anticoagulated, many of whom go on to develop fatal cerebral herniation syndromes (31). The occlusion of the internal jugular vein and the potential propagation of an intracranial venous sinus thrombus is a major reason for avoiding the placement of central venous catheters in this location among patients with acquired brain injury who are at risk for a herniation event (32).

TYPES OF HERNIATION SYNDROMES

Patients who develop unchecked intracranial compartmentalized pressures from acquired brain injury may show clinical or radiographic changes indicating an ongoing or imminent cerebral herniation syndrome (7). An awareness of how increased ICP and poor intracranial compliance manifest on the clinical exam and its adjuncts is paramount to managing the patient with neurologic critical illness.

As discussed, the skull is a fixed and rigid container filled with intravascular blood, brain parenchyma, and CSF. Any increase in volume from hemorrhage, edema, or CSF is initially compensated for by displacement of blood or CSF (1,2). Herniation occurs when these compensatory mechanisms are exceeded, resulting in a variety of neurologic syndromes. An awareness of the relevant neuroanatomy of structures that are damaged when cerebral herniation occurs, either from direct compression and neuronal dysfunction or from compromise of an anatomic region's vascular supply, is helpful in understanding how these different cerebral herniation syndromes present at the bedside. The areas of the brain at most risk for sustaining injury during a herniation event lie adjacent to more rigid structures, which include the foramen magnum, the tentorium cerebelli, and the falx cerebri. The movement of brain tissue across these three areas due to the equalization of compartmentalized pressure is responsible for the clinical manifestations and consequences of cerebral herniation.

These vary, although a discussion of the reported and commonly encountered signs follows (33).

Transtentorial Herniation

Transtentorial herniation can be divided into lateral transtentorial (uncal) herniation and central transtentorial herniation. Lateral transtentorial herniation occurs when a supratentorial mass, most commonly a temporal lobe lesion, pushes the mesial temporal lobe and uncus anteriorly and downward through the tentorial opening between the ipsilateral midbrain and the tentorium. As the herniating medial temporal lobe (uncus) begins to compress the third cranial nerve, pupillary reactivity to light may become sluggish on the side ipsilateral to the compression, or the ipsilateral pupil may show an increase in baseline size with the development of anisocoria. As the midbrain is further compressed, an indentation develops in the cerebral peduncle from compression against the contralateral tentorial (Figure 4.2), referred to as Kernohan's notch (34).

In this condition, dysfunction of the cerebral peduncle on the side opposite the mass lesion results in motor paresis on the side ipsilateral to the mass lesion that can be interpreted as a false localizing sign called *Kernohan's notch phenomenon* (34). When presented with an enlarged, sluggishly reactive pupil and developing hemiparesis, the cortical lesion causing the cerebral herniation is most likely located on the side of the abnormal pupil. A reliable sign of ongoing progression of brain tissue herniation across the tentorium is the appearance of an extensor toe response on the patient's nonhemiparetic side (33). The progression of lateral transtentorial herniation then results in obtundation with motor posturing to noxious stimuli while the enlarged pupil found earlier on exam will begin to become somewhat smaller, and the contralateral pupil may fail to react to light. Without intervention, progression to coma follows (35).

Transtentorial herniation occurs with the central downward movement of the brainstem due to pressure from the supratentorial brain components. Unlike

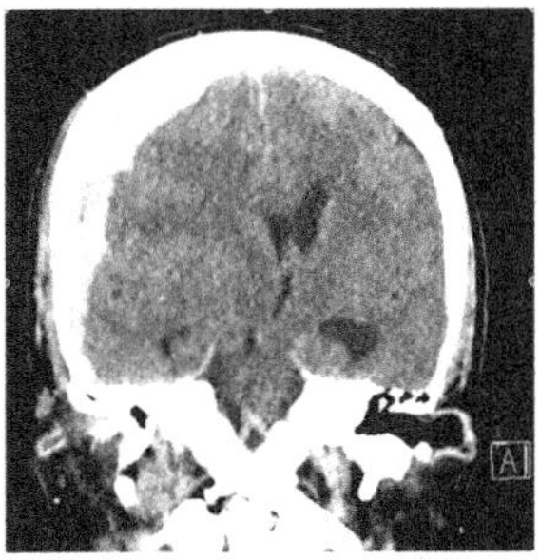

FIGURE 4.2 Coronal head CT showing Kernohan's notch phenomenon with compression of the left cerebral peduncle on the side contralateral to a right convexity subdural hematoma, resulting in right hemiparesis. A decompressive hemicraniectomy was performed with hematoma evacuation.

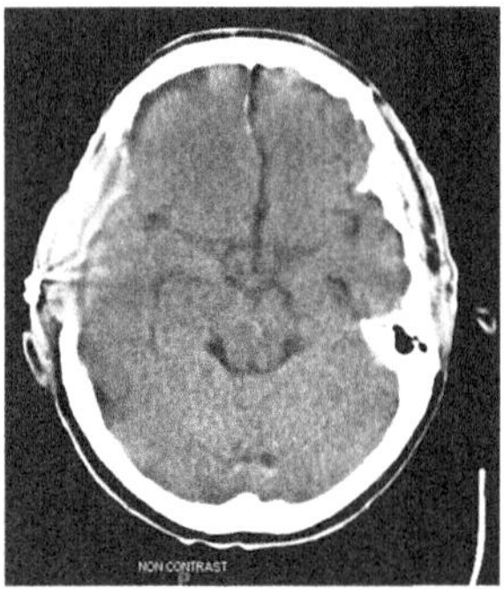

FIGURE 4.3 Axial head CT of a patient who suffered transtentorial herniation with resultant Duret hemorrhage of the midbrain.

lateral transtentorial herniation, this is more likely to occur with frontal, parietal, or occipital mass lesions rather than temporal lobe lesions. As supratentorial compartmentalized pressure increases, the midbrain is folded over onto the pons below, resulting in both neuronal injury from direct compression and the interruption of vascular supply from perforating branches of the basilar artery. This is the mechanism of vascular injury responsible for the small hemorrhages in the pons and the midbrain referred to as Duret hemorrhages (Figure 4.3) (36). Although these clearly represent a significant neurologic injury, the presence of Duret hemorrhages is not always incompatible with a good neurologic outcome (37,38).

Early clinical findings with central herniation can include subtle decreased alertness and cranial nerve palsies. There is a well-described rostral-to-caudal progression of deteriorating brainstem activity, although not all authors feel that this progression manifests clinically in such an orderly fashion (33). Pathologic yawning with intermittent deep respirations can provide early evidence of an impending herniation (35). Sixth cranial nerve palsy can occur, resulting in lateral gaze deficits and horizontal diplopia, which may be unilateral or bilateral. Extensor plantar responses and paratonia can be elicited, and a progression to somnolence with a decrease in the patient's GCS score soon follows. A nonspecific but very recognizable pattern of irregular respirations can occur, referred to as Cheyne-Stokes breathing (35). This type of breathing, noted for sustained periods of hypoventilation followed by periods of hyperventilation, has a number of causes in addition to impending cerebral herniation (39). Pressure on the tectum of the midbrain may result in a limitation of upgaze, although oculocephalic testing may be required to evaluate this in a somnolent patient (35). Motor examination is likely to show decorticate (flexor) posturing as the syndrome of central herniation progresses.

With both lateral transtentorial herniation and central herniation, posterior cerebral artery (PCA) infarctions can occur, with resultant cortical blindness.

This complication is due to the vascular compression of the PCA as it passes upward over the tentorial notch (40). These infarcts can be unilateral or bilateral, and in the setting of coma, clinical manifestations of infarct or hemorrhage in this region may be difficult to elicit. Although both types of transtentorial herniation are discussed here as separate entities, they may be less distinct from one another in actual clinical practice or at the bedside. Perhaps the most discernable difference between the two is that early in the process, lateral transtentorial herniation more often occurs with solitary unilateral pupillary dilation and a sluggish pupillary reaction to light while the patient has yet to become somnolent (33). As herniation progresses, consciousness is ultimately impaired, although recently a case of "sliding uncus syndrome" was described in which an SDH caused unilateral pupillary dilation and radiographic evidence of progressive uncal herniation with no progression to impairment in consciousness (41). After evacuation of the SDH, the patient's pupillary abnormality resolved, and his outcome was described as favorable.

Subfalcine Herniation

Subfalcine or transfalcine herniation (Figure 4.4) occurs as the brain shifts horizontally from one side to the other across the midline.

This herniation syndrome is most often seen with lateral movement, or midline shift (MLS), of one frontal lobe into the contralateral hemisphere. Based on clinical experience, subfalcine herniation is arguably the most commonly encountered herniation syndrome. This process can also be referred to as *cingulate herniation*, as this is the anatomic structure most likely to become displaced across the falx. When herniation occurs slowly, patients have a high tolerance for lateral displacement. However, when lateral movement of the

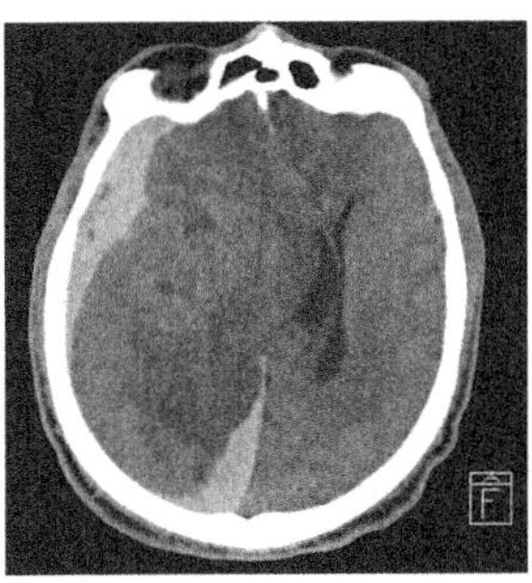

FIGURE 4.4 Axial head CT showing a subdural hematoma causing subfalcine herniation and developing cerebral ischemia.

brain occurs acutely, very small changes in horizontal displacement manifest quickly as drowsiness and later, coma. Classically, it has been reported that horizontal movement of the pineal body is well tolerated up to about 3 mm (42). Thereafter, pineal displacement of 3 to 4 mm results in drowsiness, 6 to 8.5 mm results in stupor, and 8 to 13 mm results in coma. These measurements do not necessarily reflect similar degrees of MLS at the more commonly measured level of the septum pellucidum. Recently, a bedside sonographic method for measuring and following changes by ultrasound in MLS among patients with unilateral cerebral edema or a space-occupying lesion has been described (43).

As quite a large number of patients with varying severities of intracranial pathology and any degree of MLS may show radiographic evidence of subfalcine herniation, it may not be surprising that the clinical signs of this herniation syndrome can be subtle. The most common clinical manifestations are increasing lethargy, headache, and occasionally, neurological deficits related to the compromised perfusion of one or both anterior cerebral arteries (ACA). Due to contribution to the corticospinal tracts, infarction or dysfunction of the cingulate gyrus by way of unilateral ACA compromise classically causes weakness of the contralateral lower extremity, although involvement of the proximal arm and shoulder has been reported (35). Subfalcine herniation with MLS that is progressive can lead to other syndromes, most commonly central transtentorial herniation from an unchecked mass lesion in the frontal lobe.

Cerebellar Herniation

Cerebellar or tonsillar herniation occurs from the caudal displacement of the cerebellar tonsils into the foramen magnum and the simultaneous compression of the brainstem at the level of the medulla. The tolerance for compartmentalized pressures in the cerebellum is limited, likely due to the reduced cranial volume and the proximity of vital, fiber-dense structures in the posterior fossa. It is commonly taught that processes resulting in any significant cerebellar edema, such as hemorrhage or stroke, may cause a potential neurosurgical emergency requiring a suboccipital craniectomy with a possible need for external ventricular drainage (44).

Radiographic findings of chronic tonsillar herniation are not uncommon with variations of Arnold-Chiari malformations, although very rarely complications from a Chiari malformation result in more acute presentations (45). In general, if the tonsils of the cerebellum are visible on axial images at the level of the dens, some degree of chronic or acute cerebellar herniation is present. Other processes can potentially result in tonsillar herniation, including localized CSF outflow disorders that affect the ventricular system as a whole or rarely with focal stenosis of the foramina of Magendie and Luschka (46). CSF drainage from the lumbar cistern can result in tonsillar herniation or transtentorial herniation and is reported to occur in diagnostic lumbar punctures for many conditions, including the routine evaluation of idiopathic intracranial hypertension (47). It should be emphasized that if an ongoing process can potentially result in compartmentalized posterior fossa pressure gradients, steps should be taken early to facilitate treatment prior to clinical manifestations of brainstem dysfunction. The clinical symptoms of impending cerebellar herniation are often dramatic and rapid, with hypotension, respiratory arrest, and caudal brainstem failure rapidly progressing to coma, circulatory collapse, and death. Cerebellar herniation can also manifest as a sudden death syndrome from apnea or due to dramatic hemodynamic changes from the compression of medullary respiratory and homeostatic centers. As the time to intervene may be limited, a posterior fossa hematoma or any significant fourth ventricular dilation, distortion, effacement, or obliteration from cerebellar edema of any cause requires an urgent neurosurgical evaluation for possible intervention, including suboccipital craniectomy (48). In general, medical interventions and surgical decompression should be entertained prior to the development of clinical symptoms referable to the caudal brainstem (48).

Upward Herniation

Upward herniation is the cephalad displacement of the posterior cranial fossa contents across the tentorium into the middle cranial fossa, resulting in brainstem compression (Figure 4.5).

This herniation syndrome is reported to occur with excessive CSF drainage from an external ventricular drain or shunt. The clinical presentation of upward transtentorial herniation is not consistently described, although a

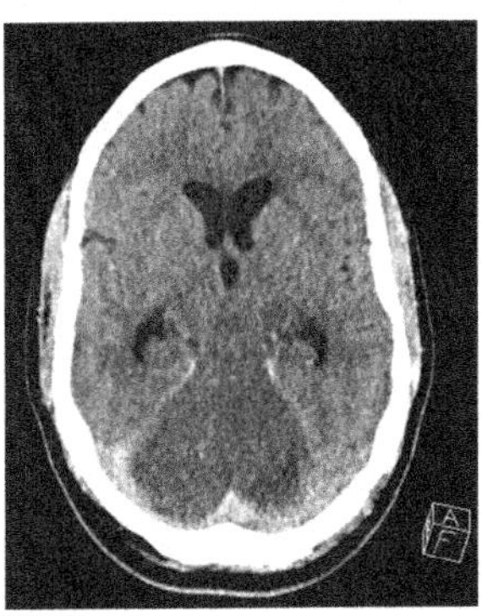

FIGURE 4.5 Axial CT of a patient with upward herniation. This image shows the development of a rounded third ventricle and hydrocephalus manifested by enlargement of the bilateral temporal horns of the lateral ventricle.

decrease in the level of consciousness and apnea have been reported during the last stages. Other reported findings are likely due to enlargement of the third ventricle after the obstruction of the cerebral aqueduct from upward herniation of the midbrain across the tentorium. The clinical manifestations of third ventricular hydrocephalus include Parinaud's syndrome—impaired upgaze, convergence-retraction nystagmus, eyelid retraction, and impaired pupillary light reflexes with the preservation of pupillary accommodation (26). Upward herniation is often best appreciated radiographically on sagittal plane images.

Paradoxical Herniation

A less commonly reported herniation syndrome is paradoxical herniation, also referred to as *low pressure herniation* or *sinking flap syndrome* (49). This is described based on the setting in which herniation occurs rather than anatomic landmarks. Reports of paradoxical herniation usually describe lumbar cistern drainage, either via a lumbar puncture or a lumbar catheter, performed in the setting of a prior craniectomy (49). Perhaps counterintuitively, this herniation syndrome manifests from the caudal movement of brain parenchyma in the setting of globally reduced ICP (50). In common with other herniation syndromes, the presence of compartmentalized pressure gradients results in cerebral displacement and herniation. If a lumbar puncture precipitated the herniation event, an emergent blood patch has been reported to reverse it (51). An awareness of this herniation syndrome is important in the management of patients who are recovering from a craniectomy. Paradoxical herniation can also occur in the setting of severe hypernatremia from diabetes insipidus, when an unchecked elevation in serum sodium causes a rapid reduction in brain volume.

Extracranial Herniation

Extracranial herniation represents a potential complication from the surgical decompression of an intracranial mass lesion where brain tissue breeches through the surgical skull defect. As with paradoxical herniation, this syndrome is described based on the setting in which herniation occurs. Most commonly, this is clinically encountered after a craniectomy as the brain parenchyma fungates through the craniotomy defect. Extracranial herniation is also seen in a severe penetrating or blunt TBI in which gross herniation of brain matter occurs through an open skull fracture. After decompressive craniectomy, extracranial herniation is reported to occur in up to 17% of patients and may represent the therapeutic decompression of intracranial hypertension (52). Unfortunately, in the setting of malignant cerebral edema, complications of extracranial

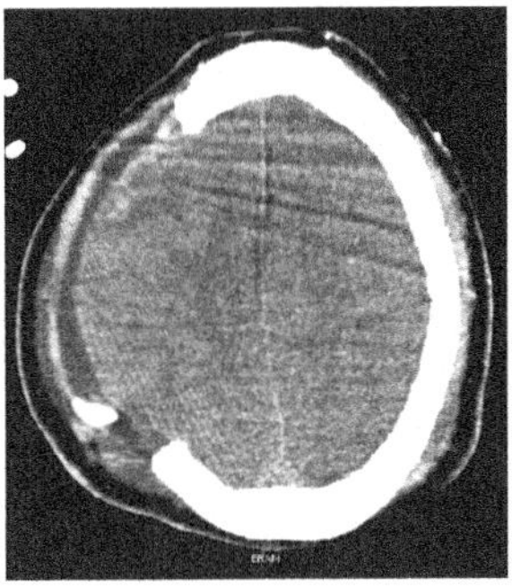

FIGURE 4.6 CT showing extracranial herniation through a surgical skull defect. This patient suffered from immune reconstitution syndrome with malignant cerebral edema treated with decompressive hemicraniectomy.

herniation can also manifest to include hemorrhagic venous infarctions and cerebral cortex lacerations. Some authors have reported that larger craniectomy defects (Figure 4.6) reduce complications from extracranial herniation (53).

THE LONG-TERM OUTCOME OF CEREBRAL HERNIATION

The classic teaching is that the outcome after a clinical cerebral herniation event is uniformly poor (35,54). With aggressive management, including both medical and surgical interventions, reasonable outcomes after cerebral herniation are well described, however. The likelihood for more favorable outcomes increases when subtle clinical or early radiographic evidence of cerebral herniation is recognized and treated. Therefore, early recognition remains paramount. The sliding uncus syndrome discussed earlier, in which clinical signs of uncal herniation are managed early and aggressively, best illustrates this point (41).

Other authors have continued to challenge the nihilism that has surrounded the discussion of outcomes after cerebral herniation. In a review by Qureshi et al, 28 patients with various neurologic disorders, including brain tumors, TBI, stroke, SAH, and ICH, had 32 episodes of clinical herniation and underwent medical reversal. Of these, 13 survived to hospital discharge (54). In this series, herniation was defined appropriately as a decrease in the patient's level of consciousness with dilation and the loss of reactivity to light of one or both pupils. Patients were treated with a stepwise sequence of actions, including endotracheal intubation, hyperventilation, and osmotic therapy, followed by the consideration of surgical decompression. The presence of bilateral nonreactive pupils, lack of surgical treatment, or repeat herniation events did not preclude the possibility of a good outcome. The presence of Duret hemorrhages in the midbrain on postherniation imaging, however, was not consistent with survival. At a mean follow-up of 11 months, seven out of the 28 patients were functionally independent. This study suggests that aggressive medical treatment of transtentorial herniation may result in good long-term functional outcome, although mortality remains high overall (54).

Others have reported subsequent series and cases of patients whose outcome after treatment of a herniation syndrome, typically transtentorial herniation, was unexpected. A large series of patients treated with 23.4% hypertonic saline for transtentorial herniation found that 32% of the cohort survived to hospital discharge. However, the short-term outcomes were less favorable, with most patients surviving with severe disability (55). Nonetheless, a recurring theme exists in the limited literature on this subject: Young patients tend to have better outcomes after transtentorial herniation than older patients, and early recognition of the event with an algorithmic approach to treatment improves both short- and long-term outcomes (56–61). Very little data is available to guide a prognosis with respect to improvement in long-term outcome after the reversal of other herniation syndromes.

MONITORING FOR IMPENDING HERNIATION

The rapid assessment of impending herniation and the employment of medical and possibly surgical interventions is the goal of therapy for patients with poor intracranial compliance and neurologic critical illness (59). Likely the best indicator of worsening neurologic status, and certainly the one most studied, is the bedside clinical examination that trained nurses and providers perform. Adjuncts to the examination may assist in predicting neurologic deterioration and herniation syndromes prior to the development of typical clinical findings. A number of adjunctive metrics have been described, including automated pupillometry, transcranial Doppler (TCD) ultrasound, electroencephalography (EEG), quantitative ICP waveform analysis, and heart rate variability.

Pupillometry

Automated pupillometry, increasingly used in the NCCU, has been studied in terms of its accuracy and ability to predict neurologic worsening in patients with TBI. This tool provides an objective measure of the size of the pupil, the percentage change in the pupil aperture when the light reflex is tested, constriction velocity, and an assessment of pupillary asymmetry. This device's utility and effectiveness at detecting early pupillary changes and the absolute presence or absence of pupillary light reflexes is reported to be greater than that of the clinical examination (62–64). The pupillometer also has greater interobserver reliability than does manual examination of the pupil's response to light (62,63). This technology's ability to predict early pupillary changes that may herald worsening intracranial compliance has also been studied. A reduction of the pupil size by less than 10% is strongly associated with an ICP greater than 20 mmHg (65). Recent reviews of pupillometry in the ICU have advocated for its use to accurately measure pupil size and reactivity and perhaps most importantly, to obtain prognostic data when an awareness of the absolute presence or absence of the pupillary light reflex is vital (66,67).

Transcranial Doppler and Pulsatility Index

TCD is a portable and noninvasive tool that is highly utilized in the NCCU. TCD monitoring is often performed on patients with aneurysmal SAH, but its use extends to other types of neurologic critical illness (68–70). TCD is widely used in the assessment of cerebral blood flow. The pulsatility index (PI), which is calculated from TCD data, can provide an estimate of intracranial compliance and a noncontinuous approximation of ICP (71). Some authors have reported that an ipsilateral-to-contralateral PI ratio greater than 1.25 is suspicious for compartmentalized ICP and mass effect, which can promote the development of herniation syndromes. An interesting study utilized TCD to evaluate patients who had sustained mild-to-moderate TBI. These patients showed little or no evidence of injury on an admission head CT, while TCD demonstrated that patients who later developed secondary neurologic deterioration up to 1 week after injury had reduced cerebral blood flow velocities (CBFV) on admission (72). Nonetheless, the use of TCD and PI as surrogates for invasive ICP measurement and to assess the risk for cerebral herniation requires further study and has not been widely implemented in clinical practice (73,74).

Optic Nerve Sheath Diameter

Another ultrasound tool that is useful in assessing patients with compromised intracranial compliance is the optic nerve sheath diameter measurement (ONSD). In patients with a consistently elevated ICP, the ONSD will reliably increase due to its relationship with the CSF compartment. Ultrasonography is performed using a linear array probe placed on the superior and lateral aspect of the orbit against the upper eyelid. This method can reliably measure the ONSD with the eye closed and angled slightly caudally and medially (75–77). For detecting an ICP greater than 20 mmHg, an ONSD greater than 0.48 cm has been found to have a sensitivity of 95% and a specificity of 93% (75). ONSD measurements, however, may not reliably reflect intermittent fluctuations in ICP, which are important in the development of herniation syndromes (78). The use of ONSD in assessing intracranial pathology is the subject of multiple ongoing clinical trials. ONSD measurement currently lacks a clearly defined role in the prediction of cerebral herniation.

Electroencephalography

The use of EEG to predict neurologic decline makes clinical sense. Many neurologists and neurosurgeons use EEG on a day-to-day basis to gauge the future risk of neurologic deterioration for patients with epilepsy. EEG changes can signal alterations in cerebral perfusion and hypoxia that may precede changes in the clinical examination or other markers of progressive cerebral edema (79). These findings can be subtle, but noting increasing or developing asymmetric slowing between hemispheres on continuous EEG, especially later progression to more obvious signs such as focal burst-suppression patterns, has been reported to predict subsequent cerebral herniation by several hours (79). The Neurocritical Care Society describes EEG as a tool for the noninvasive assessment of cerebral oxygenation and ischemia, which can precede cerebral herniation syndromes (80).

HEART RATE VARIABILITY AND INTRACRANIAL PRESSURE

The classic vital sign changes associated with cerebral herniation are well known and referred to eponymously as Cushing's triad (81). Cushing described the vasomotor changes in preclinical models of increased ICP, in which intracranial hypertension resulted in compensatory bradycardia, hyperventilation, and an increase in arterial blood pressure. These hemodynamic changes were presumed to be a physiologic compensation to ensure perfusion to the medulla. Interestingly, Cushing also reported that when the rise in ICP occurred very slowly, the "primary quickening of pulse and respiration may be absent" (81,82). In other words, the earliest indication of a departure from normal intracranial compliance was heralded not by bradycardia but by tachycardia and hyperventilation. As such, the earliest vital sign to change, as has been described for over 110 years, is the heart rate. Critically ill patients with brain injuries who develop unexplained tachycardia may warrant an evaluation for impending herniation and worsening intracranial compliance.

Other authors have described more specific changes in heart rate and electrocardiographic abnormalities associated with intracranial hypertension. Quantitative assessments of low heart rate variability have been found in association with elevation in ICP, cerebral hypoperfusion, and increased mortality in patients with head trauma (83–85). The use of heart rate variability and pulse pressure variability has also been shown to predict elevation in ICP, impending progression to brain death, and functional outcome (86). The use of this technology has not yet been widely adopted, although its noninvasive nature is appealing for selecting those patients who may require more invasive monitoring to predict clinical neurologic deterioration and herniation.

CONCLUSION

Accurately predicting patients most at risk of neurologic deterioration is a goal of neurocritical care physicians. Caring individually for patients might improve outcomes and would ultimately lead to a potential decrease in unnecessary complications from invasive management. Analyzing trend data compiled from ICP, blood pressure, and cerebral perfusion pressure may be the best way to individualize care, as has been recently proposed (67). It has been suggested that physicians consider ICP not as a target for therapy in and of itself but as a marker of underlying processes that require treatment; they should also consider intracranial compliance—rather than ICP—when attempting to individualize treatment goals (67). The degree of ICP response to noxious stimulation, ICP changes after the brief cessation of ongoing CSF drainage, or analysis of the ICP waveform may indicate compliance (Figure 4.1). The estimation of intracranial compliance may improve methods for managing and preventing the potentially devastating consequences of cerebral herniation. This practice has been aptly termed *herniation tuning* and represents a valuable area for future study (67).

Disclaimer

The opinions and views expressed herein belong solely to the authors. They are not nor should they be implied as being endorsed by the Uniformed Services University of the Health Sciences, the U.S. Army, the U.S. Air Force, the U.S. Department of Defense, or any other branch of the federal government of the United States.

References

1. Monro A. Observations on the structure and function of the nervous system. Edinburgh. 1783.

2. Kellie G. An account of the appearances observed in the dissection of two of three individuals presumed to have perished in the storm of the 3rd, and whose bodies were discovered in the vicinity of Leith on the morning of the 4th, November 1821; with some reflections of the pathology of the brain. *Trans Med Chir Soc Edinb.* 1824;1:84–169.

3. American College of Surgeons. *Advanced Trauma Life Support* (ATLS). 9th ed. Chicago: American College of Surgeons, 2012.

4. Teasdale G JB. Assessment of coma and impaired consciousness: a practical scale. *Lancet*. 1974;2:81–84.

5. Surgical management of penetrating brain injury. *J Trauma*. 2001;51(suppl 2):S16–S25.

6. Perel P, Arango M, Clayton T, et al. Predicting outcome after traumatic brain injury: practical prognostic models based on large cohort of international patients. *British Medical Journal*. 2008;336:425–429.

7. Carhuapoma J, Qureshi AI, Bhardwaj A, et al. Interhemispheric intracranial pressure gradients in massive cerebral infarction. *J Neurosurg Anesthesiol*. 2002;14(4):299–303.

8. Saehle T, Eide PK. Intracranial pressure monitoring in pediatric and adult patients with hydrocephalus and tentative shunt failure: a single-center experience over 10 years in 146 patients. *J Neurosurg*. 2015;122(5):1076–1086.

9. Balser D, Farooq S, Mehmood T, Reyes M, Samadani U. Actual and projected incidence rates for chronic subdural hematomas in United States Veterans Administration and civilian populations. *J Neurosurg*. 2015; 20:1–7.

10. Ledic D, Girotto D, Pal S, et al. Risk factors for subdural bleeding in elderly population. *Coll Antropol*. 2014;38(4):1195–1198.

11. Tanaka T, Kato N, Haseqawa Y, et al. Unpredicted sudden death due to recurrent infratentorial hemangiopericytoma presenting as massive intratumoral hemorrhage: a case report and review of the literature. *Case Rep Neurol Med*. 2014. Article ID 230681, 5 pages. http://dx.doi.org/10.1155/2014/230681.

12. McPhail M, Kriese S, Heneghan MA. Current management of acute liver failure. *Curr Opin Gastroenterol*. 2015;31(3):209–214.

13. Richardson D, Bellamy M. Intracranial hypertension in acute liver failure. *Nephrol Dial Transplant*. 2002;17(1):23–27.

14. Larson F, Gottstein J, Blei AT. Cerebral hyperemia and nitric oxide synthase in rats with ammonia-induced brain edema. *J Hepatol*. 2001;34(4):548–554.

15. Boscan P, Pina-Crespo JC, Dalo NL. Ketamine reduces lethality on the acute ammonia intoxication in mice. *Invest Clin*. 1996;37(2):129–135.

16. Cauli O, Rodrigo R, Boix J, et al. Acute liver failure-induced death of rats is delayed or prevented by blocking NMDA receptors in brain. *Am J Physiol Gastrointest Liver Physiol*. 2008;295(3):503–511.

17. Frontera J. Metabolic encephalopathies in the critical care unit. *Continuum*. 2012;18(3): 611–639.

18. Lopez-Almaraz E, Correa-Rotter R. Dialysis disequilibrium syndrome and other treatment complications of extreme uremia: a rare occurrence yet not vanished. *Hemodial Int*. 2008;12(3):301–306.

19. Osgood M, Compton R, Carandang R, et al. Rapid unexpected brain herniation in association with renal replacement therapy in acute brain injury: caution in the neurocritical care unit. *Neurocrit Care*. 2015;22(2):176–183.

20. Gordon D, Hosu L, Agabegi S, et al. Brain herniation due to syndrome of inappropriate antidiuretic hormone secretion (SIADH) after posterior spine fusion. *Paediatr Anaesth*. 2013;23(9):875–876.

21. Svensson P, Bergqvist PB, Juul KV, et al. Desmopressin in treatment of haematological disorders and in prevention of surgical bleeding. *Blood Rev*. 2014;28(3):95–102.

22. Oh J, Shin JI. Syndrome of inappropriate antidiuretic hormone secretion and cerebral/renal salt wasting syndrome: similarities and differences. *Front Pediatr*. 2015;22(2):146.

23. Marshall S, Riechers RG. Diagnosis and management of moderate and severe traumatic brain injury sustained in combat. *Mil Med.* 2012;177(suppl 8):76–85.

24. Igari Y, Hosoya T, Hayashizaki Y, et al. Sudden death due to a cystic lesion in the cerebellum. *Forensic Sci Int.* 2014;245:e25–e28.

25. El-Gaidi M, El-Nasr AH, Eissa EM. Infratentorial complications following preresection CSF diversion in children with posterior fossa tumors. *J Neurosurg Pediatr.* 2015;15(1): 4–11.

26. Antes S, Eymann R, Schmitt M, et al. Pathophysiology of brainstem lesions due to overdrainage. *Acta Neurochir Suppl.* 2012;113:117–180.

27. Ebke M, Jürgens KU, Tomandl B, et al. Surgical treatment of space occupying edema and hemorrhage due to cerebral venous thrombosis during pregnancy. *Neurocrit Care.* 2011;15(1):166–169.

28. Wijdicks E. *The Practice of Emergency and Critical Care Neurology.* Oxford: Oxford University Press; 2010.

29. Sahin N, Solak A, Genc B, et al. Cerebral venous thrombosis as a rare cause of subarachnoid hemorrhage: case report and literature review. *Clin Imaging.* 2014;38(4):373–379.

30. Yamamoto J, Kakeda S, Takahashi M, et al. Severe subarachnoid hemorrhage associated with cerebral venous thrombosis in early pregnancy: a case report. *J Emerg Med.* 2013;45(6): 849–855.

31. Lobo S, Ferro JM, Barinagarrementeria F, et al. ISCVT investigators. Shunting in acute cerebral venous thrombosis: a systematic review. *Cerebrovasc Dis.* 2014;37(1):38–42.

32. Ziai W, Chandolu S, Geocadin RG. Cerebral herniation associated with central venous catheter insertion: risk assessment. *J Crit Care.* 2013;28(2):189–195.

33. Ropper A, Samules MA, Klein JP. *Adams and Victor's Principles of Neurology.* 10th ed. China: McGraw-Hill; 2014.

34. Safavi-Abbasi S, Maurer AJ, Archer JB, et al. From the notch to a glioma grading system: the neurological contributions of James Watson Kernohan. *Neurosurg Focus.* 2014; 36(4):E4.

35. Brazis PW, Masdeu JC, Biller J. *Localization in Clinical Neurology.* Philadelphia, PA: Lippincott Williams and Wilkins; 2011.

36. Chew K, Baber Y, Iles L, et al. Duret hemorrhage: demonstration of ruptured paramedian pontine branches of the basilar artery on minimally invasive, whole body postmortem CT angiography. *Forensic Sci Med Pathol.* 2012;8(4):436–440.

37. Stiver SI GAD, Manley GT. Survival with good outcome after cerebral herniation and Duret hemorrhage caused by traumatic brain injury. *J Neurosurg.* 2009;110:1242–1246.

38. Ishizaka S, Shimizu T, Ryu N. Dramatic recovery after severe descending transtentorial herniation-induced Duret haemorrhage: a case report and review of literature. *Brain Inj.* 2014;28(3):374–377.

39. Daek M, Kirsch DB. Sleep-disordered breathing in neurologic conditions. *Clin Chest Med.* 2014;35(3):547–556.

40. Blumenfeld H, Manley GT. *Neuroanatomy Through Clinical Cases.* Sunderland, MA: Sinauer Associates; 2011.

41. Katzir M, Attia M, Sviri GE, et al. Uncal herniation in a fully conscious patient—the sliding uncus syndrome. *Br J Neurosurg.* 2014:1–2.

42. Ropper A. Lateral displacement of the brain and level of consciousness in patients with an acute hemispheral mass. *N Engl J Med.* 1986;314(15):953–958.

43. Motuel J, Biette I, Srairi M, et. Assessment of brain midline shift using sonography in neurosurgical ICU patients. *Crit Care.* 2014;18(6):676.

44. Witsch J, Neugebauer H, Zweckberger K, et al. Primary cerebellar haemorrhage: complications, treatment and outcome. *Clin Neurol Neurosurg.* 2013;115(7):863–869.

45. Meeker J, Amerine J, Kropp D, et al. The impact of Chiari malformation on daily activities: a report from the national Conquer Chiari Patient Registry database. *Disabil Health J.* 2015;8(4): 521–526.

46. Karachi C, Le Guérinel C, Brugières P, et al. Hydrocephalus due to idiopathic stenosis of the foramina of Magendie and Luschka. Report of three cases. *J Neurosurg.* 2003;98(4): 897–902.

47. Hoffman K, Chan SW, Hughes AR, et al. Management of cerebellar tonsillar herniation following lumbar puncture in idiopathic intracranial hypertension. *Case Rep Crit Care.* Volume 2015 (2015). Article ID 895035, 4 pages. http://dx.doi.org/10.1155/2015/895035.

48. Bullock MR, Chesnut R, Ghajar J, et al. Surgical management of traumatic parenchymal lesions. *Neurosurgery.* 2006;58(suppl 3):S25–S46.

49. Zhao J, Li G, Zhang Y, et al. Sinking skin flap syndrome and paradoxical herniation secondary to lumbar drainage. *Clin Neurol Neurosurg.* 2015;133: 6–10.

50. Vilela MD. Delayed paradoxical herniation after a decompressive craniectomy: case report. *Surg Neurol.* 2008;69:293–296.

51. Muehlschlegel S, Voetsch B, Sorond FA. Emergent epidural blood patch: lifesaving treatment of paradoxical herniation. *Arch Neurol.* 2009;66:670–671.

52. Saade N, Veiga JC, Cannoni LF, et al. Evaluation of prognostic factors of decompressive craniectomy in the treatment of severe traumatic brain injury. *Rev Col Bras Cir.* 2014;41(4): 256–262.

53. Yang XF, Wen L, Shen F, et al. Surgical complications secondary to decompressive craniectomy in patients with a head injury: a series of 108 consecutive cases. *Acta Neurochir* (Wien). 2008;150:1241–1247.

54. Qureshi A, Geocadin RG, Suarez JI, et al. Long-term outcome after medical reversal of transtentorial herniation in patients with supratentorial mass lesions. *Crit Care Med.* 2000;28(5):1556–1564.

55. Koenig MA, Bryan M, Lewin JL III, et al. Reversal of transtentorial herniation with hypertonic saline. *Neurology.* 2008;70:1023–1029.

56. Hirsch K, Spock T, Koenig MA, et al. Treatment of elevated intracranial pressure with hyperosmolar therapy in patients with renal failure. *Neurocrit Care.* 2012;17(3):388–394.

57. Ratnasingam D, Lovick DS, Weber DM, et al. An unusual recovery from traumatic brain injury in a young man. *Linacre Q.* 2015;82(1):55–66.

58. Yeo S, Jang SH. Corticospinal tract recovery in a patient with traumatic transtentorial herniation. *Neural Regen Res.* 2013;8(5):469–473.

59. Qureshi AI SJI. More evidence supporting a brain code protocol for reversal of transtentorial herniation. *Neurology.* 2008;70:990–991.

60. Yamahata H, Hirabaru M, Arita K. Rapid spontaneous resolution of neurological signs and cerebral herniation caused by intracerebral hemorrhage—case report. *Neurol Med Chir* (Tokyo). 2010;50(5):390–392.

61. Acakpo-Satchivi L, Luerssen TG. Brain herniation through an internal subdural membrane: a rare complication seen with chronic subdural hematomas in children [case report]. *J Neurosurg.* 2007;107(suppl 6):485–488.

62. Meeker M, Du R, Baccheti P, et al. Pupil examination: validity and clinical utility of an automated pupillometer. *J Neurosci Nurs.* 2005;37(1):34–40.

63. Yan S, Tu Z, Lu W, et al. Clinical utility of an automated pupillometer for assessing and monitoring recipients of liver transplantation. *Liver Transpl.* 2009;15(12):1718–1727.

64. Larson M, Muhludeen I. Pupillometric analysis of the "absent light reflex." *Arch Neurol.* 1995;52(4):369–372.

65. Taylor W, Chen JW, Meltzer H, et al. Quantitative pupillometry, a new technology: normative data and preliminary observations in patients with acute head injury [technical note]. *J Neurosurg.* 2003;98(1):205–213.

66. Sahar F, Suarez JL. Automated pupillometer for monitoring the critically ill patient: a critical appraisal. *J Crit Care.* 2014;29(4):599–603.

67. Chesnut R. A conceptual approach to managing severe traumatic brain injury in a time of uncertainty. *Ann N Y Acad Sci.* 2015;1345(1):99–107.

68. Marshall SA, Nyquist P, Ziai WC. The role of transcranial Doppler ultrasonography in the diagnosis and management of vasospasm after aneurysmal subarachnoid hemorrhage. *Neurosurg Clin N Am.* 2010;21(2):291–303.

69. Razumovsky A, Tigno T, Hochheimer SM, et al. Cerebral hemodynamic changes after wartime traumatic brain injury. *Acta Neurochir Suppl.* 2013;115:87–90.

70. Marshall S, Kalanuria A, Markandaya M, et al. The management of intracerebral pressure in the neurosciences critical care unit. *Neurosurg Clin N Am.* 2013;24(3):361–373.

71. Brandi G, Béchir M, Sailer S, et al. Transcranial color-coded duplex sonography allows to assess cerebral perfusion pressure noninvasively following severe traumatic brain injury. *Acta Neurochir* (Vienna). 2010;152(6):965–972.

72. Bouzat P, Francony G, Declety P, et al. Transcranial Doppler to screen on admission patients with mild to moderate traumatic brain injury. *Neurosurgery.* 2011;68(6):1603–1609.

73. Zweifel C, Czosnyka M, Carrera E, et al. Reliability of the blood flow velocity pulsatility index for assessment of intracranial and cerebral perfusion pressures in head-injured patients. *Neurosurgery.* 2012;71(4):853–861.

74. de Riva N, Budohoski KP, Smielewski P, et al.Transcranial Doppler pulsatility index: what it is and what it isn't. *Neurocrit Care.* 2012;17(58–66).

75. Rajajee V, Vanaman M, Fletcher JJ, et al. Optic nerve ultrasound for the detection of raised intracranial pressure. *Neurocrit Care.* 2011;15(3):506–515.

76. Amini A, Kariman H, Arhami Dolatabadi A, et al. Use of the sonographic diameter of optic nerve sheath to estimate intracranial pressure. *Am J Emerg Med.* 2013;31(1):236–239.

77. Moretti R, Pizzi B, Cassini F, et al. Reliability of optic nerve ultrasound for the evaluation of patients with spontaneous intracranial hemorrhage. *Neurocrit Care.* 2009;11(3):406–410.

78. Rajajee V FJ, Rochlen LR, Jacobs TL. Comparison of accuracy of optic nerve ultrasound for the detection of intracranial hypertension in the setting of acutely fluctuating vs stable intracranial pressure: post-hoc analysis of data from a prospective, blinded single center study. *Crit Care.* 2012;16(3): R79.

79. Newey C, Sarwal A, Hantus S. Continuous electroencephalography (cEEG) changes precede clinical changes in a case of progressive cerebral edema. *Neurocrit Care.* 2013;18(2):261–265.

80. Le Roux P, Menon DK, Citerio G, et al. The international multidisciplinary consensus conference on multimodality monitoring in neurocritical care: evidentiary tables: a statement for healthcare professionals from the neurocritical care society and the European society of intensive care medicine. *Neurocrit Care.* 2014;21(suppl 2):297–361.

81. Cushing H. Some experimental and clinical observations concerning states of increased intracranial tension. *Am J Med Sco.* 1902;124:375–400.

82. Koehler P, Bruyn GW, Pearce JMS. *Neurologic Eponyms.* New York, NY: Oxford University Press; 2000.

83. Katsanos AH1 KP, Tsivgoulis G, Kyritsis AP, et al. Electrocardiographic abnormalities and cardiac arrhythmias in structural brain lesions. *Int J Cardiol.* 2013;167(2):328–334.

84. Kox M, Vrouwenvelder MQ, Pompe JC, et al. The effects of brain injury on heart rate variability and the innate immune response in critically ill patients. *J Neurotrauma.* 2012;29(5): 747–755.

85. Mowery N, Norris PR, Riordan W, et al. Cardiac uncoupling and heart rate variability are associated with intracranial hypertension and mortality: a study of 145 trauma patients with continuous monitoring. *J Trauma.* 2008;65(3):621–627.

86. Kahraman S, Dutton RP, Hu P, et al. Heart rate and pulse pressure variability are associated with intractable intracranial hypertension after severe traumatic brain injury. *J Neurosurg Anesthesiol.* 2010;22(4):296–302.

5

Osmotic Agents for the Treatment of Intracranial Hypertension and Cerebral Edema

Julia C. Durrant
Holly E. Hinson

CASE STUDY *A 20-year-old male driving 40 miles per hour rear-ended a large truck while distracted by texting on his cell phone. His Glasgow Coma Scale (GCS) score was 4 on the scene. He was intubated prior to his arrival to the hospital. On admission, he was comatose, with closed eyes. His pupils were midsize and sluggishly reactive, and corneal reflexes were present, as well as a cough to deep suctioning. He had no gag reflex. Noxious stimulation produced extensor posturing on the right side with no movement noted on the left. CT imaging of the head revealed bilateral frontal contusions and small frontal subdural and diffuse subarachnoid hemorrhages. A subarachnoid intracranial monitor (bolt) was placed. Initial continuous readings registered an intracranial pressure (ICP) of 15 mmHg, which steadily rose to 28 mmHg in the next 12 hours. The pupils became slightly more oval shaped, with a reduced reaction to light. Serum sodium was 139 mEq/L.*

INTRODUCTION AND HISTORICAL PERSPECTIVES

The medical management of intracranial hypertension and cerebral herniation consists of reducing intracranial vault contents through a variety of strategies, including the reduction of arterial and venous blood, the decompression of mass lesions, the drainage of cerebrospinal fluid (CSF), and the reduction of brain tissue edema. This chapter focuses on the osmotherapeutic management of increased ICP through the reduction of cerebral edema, while subsequent chapters in this book will focus on other interventions often employed simultaneously or in an algorithmic escalation.

The discovery of the use of osmotic agents to decrease cerebral edema was inadvertent. In 1919 Lewis Weed and Paul McKibben, research fellows at Johns Hopkins University, injected hypertonic solutions of sodium chloride into the veins of cats in an attempt to measure the amount of salt transported from blood to the CSF (1). They quickly noted that shortly after injection, they were unable to obtain fluid from the subarachnoid space. Following this observation, they attached a manometer to the needle and measured the pressure changes to the spinal fluid following intravenous (IV) injections of solutions of varying tonicity. A "marked and sustained rise" in the pressure of the CSF was noted after the injection of distilled water, while IV injections of hypertonic solutions (concentrated sodium chloride, sodium bicarbonate, sodium sulfate, and glucose) revealed a marked and rapid fall in the pressure measurements. Next, they performed craniotomies to permit direct visualization of the cranial vault and observed shrinkage of the brain with hypertonic solutions and inversely, "protrusion and herniation of the brain" with the administration of hypotonic solutions. These observations laid the foundation for the concept of osmotherapy and were soon implemented into research and clinical practice (2–5).

Early forays into osmotherapy included the use of IV hypertonic (50%) glucose (6), dextrose (2), or sucrose (4); however, their use was limited by a rebound in ICP and with sucrose, the occurrence of acute tubular necrosis and crystalluria (7). Likewise, experimentation with human plasma proteins, while effective at reducing ICPs, was limited due to allergic reactions and the cost of preparation (8,9). Due to these complications, the use of hyperosmolar agents fell out of favor in the management of brain swelling and hydrocephalus during the 1930s (3) and would not be explored again for another 20 years.

The 1950s saw a renewed interest in hyperosmolar agents for the management of cerebral edema. Urea, developed as a diuretic, was the first osmotic agent to receive widespread use after multiple animal experiments demonstrated an efficacy in reducing brain volume and pressure (10–12). By the 1960s, it was considered a standard of care for neurosurgical patients. Unfortunately, difficulties in preparing the IV infusion, as well as concerns about unpredictable rebound ICP, acute renal failure in dehydrated patients, and platelet dysfunction in patients with intracranial hemorrhages, rapidly limited its use. The sugar alcohols mannitol and glycerol had fewer side effects and eventually replaced other osmotherapeutics.

PRINCIPLES OF OSMOTHERAPY

The determinants of osmolality, the concentration of solutes (osm) per kilogram (kg) of solvent of plasma in normal, healthy subjects are sodium salts (chloride and bicarbonate), glucose, and urea (13). Osmolality can be measured in a laboratory with the use of an osmometer to measure the depression of the freezing point of the plasma. In normal subjects, plasma osmolality is approximately 285 to 290 mOsm/kg, although the reference range can vary depending on the laboratory. Osmolarity is a formula representing the solutes, which under ordinary circumstances contribute nearly all of the osmolality of the sample (14). Generally, serum osmolarity is calculated by the following equation:

$$\text{Serum osmolarity} = (2 \times \text{serum [Na]}) + [\text{glucose, in mg/dL}]/18 + [\text{blood urea nitrogen, in mg/dL}]/2.8$$

The sodium value is multiplied by 2 to account for the chloride and bicarbonate anions that circulate in the plasma. Glucose and blood urea nitrogen are divided by 18 and 2.8, respectively, to convert units of mg/dL into mmol/kg.

The difference between the measured and the calculated values is the osmole gap. The units of the measured osmolality (mOsm/kg) and calculated osmolarity (mmol/kg) are different; however, in clinical practice, the small amount of error the discrepancy introduces is negligible (15,16), and therefore the osmole gap is calculated in units of mOsm/L. Under normal circumstances, the osmole gap should be quite small, within 10 mOsm/L, as the calculated and measured osmoles should be equal. An elevation of the osmole gap suggests either a decrease in the water content of the serum from either severe hyperproteinemia or hyperlipidemia or more commonly, the presence of an unmeasured solute. Other toxic alcohols, such as methanol, ethylene glycol, and acetone can also cause an elevated osmole gap, and importantly, low molecular weight sugars such as mannitol and sorbitol also produce an elevated osmole gap, thus making an osmole gap a helpful clinical tool.

Cell membranes, in general, are freely permeable to water, allowing the passive diffusion of water while restricting the movement of other solutes. Water, therefore, will flow from body compartments with low osmolality to higher osmolality to maintain an equivalent osmolality of the intracellular, intravascular, and interstitial compartments (8). The introduction of hyperosmolar solutions into the plasma immediately draws water from adjacent tissues to dilute the plasma.

In the central nervous system, tight junctions between adjacent endothelium membranes across much of the brain parenchyma limit the passive diffusion of water. Aquaporin (AQP) channels in astrocytic end-feet connect with blood vessels and regulate brain water homeostasis (17). Water and solute transport via AQPs depends on concentration gradients across the membrane, but the number of channels in the membrane and their permeability determine the magnitude of the transportation (18). The permeability of the membranes to different solutes influences the osmotic forces between the two membranes, a concept known as *tonicity* or *effective osmolality*. Tonicity, a measurement of the effective osmotic pressure gradient that the concentration of impermeable solutes across membranes generates, depends on the properties of the separating membranes. The concentration of these solutions determines the direction and extent of diffusion. Mathematically, tonicity is expressed in the form of "osmotic reflection coefficient (σ)" of a given solute, where 0 represents a solute that exerts no osmotic force, and 1 represents a highly osmotically active solute, which strongly draws water across the membrane. Glucose, urea, or the ingestion of toxic alcohols can increase the plasma osmolality and contribute to a larger osmole gap, but as the blood-brain barrier is relatively permeable to these molecules, the osmotic gradient is smaller and less sustained compared to gradients that equal concentrations of mannitol or sodium, which are much less permeable, produce (8).

The ideal solutions used in osmotherapy contain simple solutes of low molecular weight, have hyperosmolar concentrations relative to plasma, and have osmotic reflection coefficients that approach 1. Neurological diseases and injuries can disrupt the impermeability of the blood-brain barrier, which can alter the coefficient effect in vivo. The volume of undamaged brain tissue appears to influence the efficacy of the hyperosmolar agents (19,20). Urea and glycerol are examples of low-tonicity agents ($\sigma = 0.59$ and 0.48, respectively): They contribute to the measured osmolality of the serum, but as they easily diffuse across cell membranes, water concentrations are unchanged, and the osmotic pressure gradient is low (15). The σ of mannitol equals 0.9 while sodium chloride approaches 1 in physiological states. Osmotherapy agents must have both a high reflection coefficient and an osmolality above the normal serum value of approximately 287 mOsm/L to be effective in reducing intracranial hypertension and brain volume (21). Table 5.1 lists the comparative osmolality, sodium concentrations, and osmotic reflection coefficient of common IV infusion agents.

The repeated or continuous administration of hyperosmolar agents results in a sustained hyperosmolar plasma state. Water initially moves from intracellular and interstitial spaces to extracellular, causing cell and brain shrinkage; however, this effect is not permanent, and the brain adapts over a period of

TABLE 5.1 Comparison of osmolality, sodium concentration, and the osmotic reflection coefficient of common intravenous solutions

Solution	Osmolality (mOsm/L)	Sodium Concentration (mEq/L)	Reflection Coefficient (σ)
Lactated Ringer's solution	273	130	0.8
Saline 0.9%	285	154	1.0
Urea	Variable	N/A	0.59
Mannitol 20%	1,375	N/A	0.9
Saline 3%	1,026	513	1.0
Glycerol 10%	5,715	N/A	0.48
Saline 7.5%	2,566	1,283	1.0
Saline 23.4%	8,008	4,004	1.0

Source: Adapted with permission from Hinson HE, Stein D, Sheth KN. Hypertonic saline and mannitol therapy in critical care neurology. *J Intensive Care Med.* 2013;28(1):3–11.

hours. Over a short period of time, electrolytes and idiogenic osmoles, including carbohydrates, amino acids, and small proteins, gradually accumulate to counteract the dehydration effect (22–24). Maintaining a steady serum hyperosmolar state is therefore crucial to prevent a reversal in water osmosis and an increase in cerebral edema and ICP (20).

Osmotic agents: mannitol

Mannitol, a sugar alcohol, was established to reduce ICP in animal studies in the 1960s (25,26). Mannitol is metabolically inert and freely filtered by the kidney. It acts as an osmotic diuretic, facilitating the excretion of water and inhibiting the renal tubular reabsorption of sodium, chloride, and other solutes. It contributes to sustained hyperosmolarity by dehydrating brain tissues (20). With an osmotic reflection coefficient of 0.9, it has limited penetration across the blood-brain barrier. It is given in a 20% concentrated solution as an IV bolus over 20 to 30 minutes in doses that range from 0.25 to 1.5 g/kg of body weight. In situations of acute herniation, 1 g/kg is used to achieve an urgent reduction of intracranial hypertension. A reduction in ICP can be seen within 5 minutes; the peak effect on the reduction of brain volume is 15 to 35 minutes after infusion (26). The duration of its effect on ICP is variable but may last from 1.5 to 6 hours; larger doses have a more prolonged effect (8). For patients requiring a prolonged reduction in ICP, doses of 0.25 to 1 g/kg may be repeated every 2 to 6 hours (27).

The kidney rapidly clears mannitol, with an elimination half-life of approximately 30 to 60 minutes in the doses typically used in neurocritical care, depending primarily on the glomerular filtration rate (GFR), with a fall to 10% or less of the initial dose after 4 hours (28). This establishes a temporary transient osmotic gradient favoring the movement of water out of red blood cells, skeletal muscle, viscera, and the brain, as well as limiting the absorption of mannitol into interstitial tissue (8). In patients with increased total body water (eg, ascites or severe peripheral edema) mannitol will be cleared more slowly than predicted from GFR alone. Serum mannitol levels are not available commercially, making it challenging to determine when redosing of mannitol might be safe. For this reason, checking the osmole gap, as described previously, may be useful in patients with a diminished GFR. A gap falling within the normal range suggests that a patient has sufficiently eliminated the mannitol and may be redosed (16,29).

In addition to osmotic forces, mannitol exhibits other advantageous properties. Mannitol has been shown to reduce blood viscosity by shrinking the volume of the red blood cell as well as reducing adhesiveness, allowing for better cerebral blood flow at lower blood volumes (24,30), independent of hematocrit (26,31). In addition, mannitol is a known free radical scavenger (32) and inhibitor of apoptosis (33), which may have a protective effect in the microvascular circulation, in addition to the increased oxygen delivery to end organs (34). It is unclear how clinically relevant these properties are with the reduction of cerebral edema.

Mannitol also works by increasing cardiac output and blood pressure, due to the hemodilution effect of the increased extracellular and intravascular volume. When autoregulation pathways are intact, compensatory cerebral vasoconstriction occurs, leading to decreased cerebral blood volume in the intracranial vault (8,35). With impaired autoregulation, reductions in cerebral blood volume and ICP may be limited. Last, it has been postulated that the profound diuresis may contribute partially to the lessening of ICP due to the reduction in central venous pressure (CVP) and total body water (8); however, the need for adequate circulating volume to maintain cerebral perfusion pressures and the hypoviscosity of blood cells hinder the practicality of allowing diuresis without the aggressive replacement of fluids.

Administration

The administration of hyperosmotic agents may be lifesaving and should be given as timely as possible. Mannitol is a vesicant, or an agent that may cause blistering, skin sloughing, and/or tissue necrosis upon extravasation into the tissues. However, reports of significant tissue injury are limited (36). When surveyed, most neurocritical care practitioners were comfortable administering mannitol without central access (37). Careful peripheral vein selection is important. Veins that are small or fragile, in areas of flexion, or in extremities with preexisting edema or trauma should be avoided (38). In concentrations greater than 15%, mannitol can crystalize when exposed to low temperatures. The solution should be inspected for crystal formation before administration. If crystals are present, the product should be redissolved by warming the solution to 60°C and then cooling to room temperature. Because of the potential for crystal formation, mannitol must be administered through a 5-micron, in-line filter set. Mannitol may not be administered with blood products because of the risk of agglutination or clumping of red blood cells (27).

Adverse reactions

It is important to monitor patients for adverse effects that may result from the administration of mannitol. Mannitol at high doses (greater than 200 g/day) has been associated with the induction of acute renal failure. It has been postulated to occur because of altered glomerular hemodynamics: Large doses of mannitol cause increased sodium and other solute excretions that trigger afferent intrarenal vasoconstriction, in combination with intravascular volume contraction from diuresis (39). Patients at high risk for renal failure include those with preexisting chronic renal insufficiency, particularly diabetic nephropathy, sepsis, or hypovolemia, and those receiving the repeated administration of high doses of the drug. Renal function usually resolves after the discontinuation of mannitol; however, hemodialysis may be required (40,41). As described, mannitol can induce profound diuresis—a 250 mL bolus of mannitol can produce 1.5 L of urine. Up to 15% of the filtered sodium is excreted, in addition to other ions such as potassium, calcium, magnesium, phosphate, and bicarbonate (42). As elevated serum sodium levels are often a concurrent goal, practitioners may choose to administer hypertonic saline (HS) to offset the drop in serum sodium and replace the volume loss associated with mannitol administration. Urinary concentration and dilution ability is severely impaired. The close monitoring of urine output and the replacement of urine with normal saline to maintain euvolemia minimizes the risk for hemodynamic compromise and renal insufficiency (20). Repeat administration should be delayed if the osmole gap is greater than 20 (40).

Occasionally, a rapid infusion of mannitol may also cause acute hypotension, thought to be due to a decrease in systemic vascular resistance from the expansion of plasma volume (43). This is usually transient and occurs in patients who are relatively volume depleted, but as it can lead to decreased cerebral perfusion pressures, it can quickly offset any potential benefit. Additional volume replacement and vasopressor support may be needed; hypotension can be avoided by a lower rate of injection (44).

Rebound intracranial hypotension has long been a concern with the use of hyperosmotic agents, particularly mannitol, due to the accumulation of osmotic agents and water in damaged tissues with a leaky blood-brain barrier (8). Mannitol has been observed in the tissues of primary brain tumors (45,46), but the clinical relevance has been uncertain, as mannitol is not trapped metabolically in the brain and would be removed via its concentration gradient as it is excreted in the urine (24). Repeated administration without time allowed to excrete the agent or continuous infusions may contribute to rebound elevations in ICP and should be avoided.

Osmotic Agents: Hypertonic Saline

Although Weed and McKibben's initial studies on ICP were performed using injections of saline of various concentrations, HS had limited clinical use until nearly 70 years later. Several case reports were published documenting the use of HS in the treatment of resistant intracranial hypertension after traumatic brain injury (TBI) (47). HS (any concentration of sodium chloride greater than physiologic saline 0.9%) was initially used primarily for small-volume fluid resuscitation in hemorrhagic shock. Those patients who had sustained TBI and had low presenting GCS scores appeared to benefit the most from the HS (48), with higher survival rates and better outcomes. Animal models validated that HS was as effective as mannitol at reducing ICP and cerebral edema (49,50). Clinical studies confirmed it to be effective in reducing ICP, including cases in which ICP was refractory to mannitol (51–53). Gradually, HS grew in popularity as an alternative or adjuvant to mannitol.

Like mannitol, HS has multiple mechanisms of action thought to play a role in the amelioration of cerebral edema and elevated intracranial hypertension. HS optimizes the rheological properties of the blood by increasing plasma volume, reducing blood viscosity, and increasing capillary blood flow and oxygen delivery in the microcirculation (54). In concert, the HS-induced increase in intravascular volume leads to a baroreceptor-controlled vasoconstriction of cerebral arterioles that reduces cerebral blood volume and ICP when autoregulation pathways are intact (55).

Sodium's osmotic reflection coefficient (σ) equals 1 in physiological states, theoretically making it a more effective osmotic agent than mannitol, as penetration across the blood-brain barrier and the potential to cause rebound intracranial hypertension should be less (56,57). Similarly, the osmotic gradient moves water from the cerebral intracellular and interstitial spaces into the capillaries, thereby reducing cerebral water content and bulk, with less potential for rebound cerebral hypertension. HS has been demonstrated to be a potent volume expander—an infusion of HS can increase the intravascular volume by as much as four times the infused volume within minutes (58). The increased volume contributes to increased preload and increased cardiac output and does not cause profound diuresis.

Other unique extraosmotic properties may contribute to its clinical effectiveness. HS rapidly restores normal resting membrane potentials and cell volume (59,60). It decreases the formation and/or increases the resistance to reabsorption of the CSF (61). Newer models of the molecular mechanisms of cerebral edema may also provide insight into additional contributions. Animal models have demonstrated the downregulation of the expression of aquaporin-4 (AQP4) water channels after the administration of HS, which may contribute to longer-lasting antiedema effects (62,63). In addition, recent laboratory studies have suggested that HS may play a role in immune modulation, with the downregulation of proinflammatory molecules in leukocytes and neutrophils (64–66); the clinical significance of such a role remains unknown.

Administration

Authors cite numerous concentrations of HS in the literature, varying between 2% to 23.4%. Historically, it was recommended that concentrations of saline greater than 2% be given through a central venous catheter to reduce the risk of phlebitis, vein sclerosis, and venous thrombosis (60). More recently, a few trials document the use of 3% and 7.5% saline in peripheral veins with no reported phlebitis or sclerosis (67,68). Careful prospective studies of this issue are warranted. The choice of which concentration of HS to administer depends largely on the clinical situation; access type, the urgency of neurologic deterioration, volume status, and baseline serum sodium values all factor in to the decision-making process. As expected, larger volumes of less concentrated HS are required for comparable increases in serum sodium to more concentrated formulations. Lower concentrations (2%–3%) are typical of continuous infusions. In the extreme scenario of transtentorial herniation, boluses (30–60 mL) of 23.4% HS reversed 75% of clinical herniation events in a cohort of patients with mixed etiologies of acute brain injury in one retrospective case series (69).

As with mannitol, the conventional wisdom has been that bolus dosing is a superior strategy to continuously infusing HS for cerebral edema management. Clinicians worry that continuous infusions may reset the osmostat, thus pushing the threshold of efficacy closer to serum sodium values of 160 mEq/L and risking renal failure. Additionally, Qureshi et al retrospectively observed a higher mortality rate in TBI patients receiving continuous HS infusions over those who did not (70). However, several newer studies have utilized continuous infusions without complication. Hauer et al completed an open-label, prospective study in a mixed neurologic population (intracerebral hemorrhage [ICH], ischemic stroke, and aneurysmal subarachnoid hemorrhage) of continuous infusions of HS for approximately 14 days, the results of which were compared to historical controls. They observed fewer episodes of elevated ICP and an improved mortality rate in the treatment group (71). Moreover, rebound elevated ICP was not observed after discontinuation of the infusion. The same group also measured perihematoma volume in patients with ICH who received continuous HS infusions, again with historical controls, and found reduced cerebral edema in the treatment group (72). Investigators observed a similar reassuring safety profile in a retrospective cohort of TBI patients (73). None of these trials were randomized nor was bolus dosing compared head to head with continuous infusions, thus a definitive conclusion on the issue cannot be stated. Continuous infusions of HS are likely safe but may or may not be as effective as bolus dosing for cerebral edema management.

Adverse reactions

The most worrisome adverse effect from HS is central pontine myelinolysis (CPM) or osmotic demyelination syndrome, the destruction of myelinated fibers often but not exclusively in the pons after a rapid rise in serum sodium. CPM is well documented in malnourished patients with preexisting severe hyponatremia (74–76). Animal studies have demonstrated that inducing hypernatremia to levels of 145 to 155 mEq/L does not cause myelin injury in uninjured rats (77). To date, human trials have not documented the development of myelinolysis with the use of HS for elevated ICP or cerebral edema (78–81).

Oligouric acute renal failure has been reported in burn patients whose serum concentration was greater than 160 mEq/L for prolonged periods after receiving HS as a resuscitation fluid (82). Studies in the use of HS for neurological conditions have not revealed cases of acute renal failure (83–85); however, a recent retrospective analysis linked hypernatremia to the development of acute kidney failure in patients with subarachnoid hemorrhage (86). Frequent monitoring of serum sodium levels, which should not be allowed to rise above 160 mEq/L, is recommended. HS should be utilized with caution in patients with underlying organ dysfunction who are already at risk for renal issues (78).

Other potential renal effects of HS infusions include hypokalemia and hyperchloremic metabolic acidosis from the large amount of chloride, as well as from the inhibition of resorption of bicarbonate from the proximal renal tubules. Infusion mixtures of 50:50 sodium chloride-sodium acetate may ameliorate this problem (79).

In contrast to mannitol, HS causes intravascular volume expansion. This expansion can lead to cardiac depression, congestive heart failure, and even myocardial infarction (MI) in critically ill patients with multiorgan dysfunction, especially if diastolic heart failure is present (78,80). This is especially true in patients with hepatic failure with associated cerebral edema. Furosemide or other loop diuretics can be administered concurrently to mitigate this risk (20).

Second-Line Agents

Glycerol

Glycerol is another sugar alcohol utilized for the reduction of intracranial hypertension. Naturally present and metabolized in mammalian tissues, glycerol has been noted to be efficacious in both IV and oral formulations for the reduction of ICP (87,88). Glycerol produces fewer systemic side effects, and it reduces ICP promptly; however, it diffuses easily across the blood-brain barrier into the brain parenchyma and the CSF (σ=0.48), raising concerns about rebound edema (89). Brain tissue metabolism may reduce this phenomenon (87,90); studies are lacking to address this controversy. It has been postulated that glycerol may provide neuroprotection to the injured brain by providing an alternative source of energy when glucose is unavailable (91). A Cochrane review found some evidence that glycerol improves short-term survival after ischemic stroke but little evidence to determine whether glycerol helps reduce disability after stroke (92). Currently, it is still used frequently throughout Asia and some European countries and is usually administered intravenously in 10% concentrations in 500 mL normal saline over 4 hours (88,89,93,94). Side effects appear to be negligible (92).

Sorbitol

Like glycerol, sorbitol has been used infrequently to reduce intracranial hypertension, mostly in Germany (95). The usual dosage to effectively reduce ICP is 125 ml of a 40% concentration infused intravenously over 20 minutes. The effects last approximately 1 to 2 hours. Sorbitol is primarily metabolized and cleared by the liver (85%), while the other 15% is excreted in the urine; caution should be maintained in patients with liver impairment. Hyperglycemia is common after administration, particularly in patients with impaired glucose tolerance, often warranting insulin administration. Similar to glycerol, sorbitol is metabolized by brain tissue, reducing central nervous compartment accumulation and potentially reducing the risk of a rebound phenomenon (96,97).

Furosemide

Diuretics can decrease total body water, thereby increasing blood osmolality and drawing water from the cerebral tissue. Furosemide (1 mg/kg/day in divided doses), a loop diuretic, has sometimes been administered either alone or in combination with mannitol, with variable success. The main drawback of this strategy is that volume depletion may reduce cerebral perfusion pressure. For this reason, furosemide is not a first-line agent for cerebral edema management. Other diuretics, such as acetazolamide, have played a role in the treatment of idiopathic intracranial hypertension but are not recommended in the treatment of acute brain injuries (93).

DISEASE-SPECIFIC OSMOTHERAPY

The majority of the literature regarding osmotherapy and cerebral edema or ICP comes from case reports and case series from the 1990s. However, a few more recent and/or notable trials bear mentioning.

Traumatic Brain Injury

Based on early experiences with HS as a resuscitation fluid, investigators hypothesized that HS might be a superior resuscitation fluid for patients sustaining a TBI. A multicenter, randomized blinded clinical trial failed to show any differences in neurologic outcome or survival between patients receiving a single bolus of HS vs. normal saline in the field (67). Once a patient develops raised ICP from a TBI, there appears to be no one optimal osmotherapeutic choice. Although there may be a trend toward higher efficacy with HS, both mannitol and HS effectively lower raised ICP in TBI (98). Additionally, equiosmolar infusions of 8.4% sodium bicarbonate are as effective as 5% sodium chloride for the reduction of raised ICP after TBI (99). As of the 2007 edition of recommendations, the Brain Trauma Foundation guidelines only recommend mannitol for ICP reduction, citing lack of evidence, though these guidelines lag behind current practice (100).

Ischemic Stroke

Clinical evidence has not supported the theoretic concerns about worsening midline shift by drawing water out of the contralateral hemisphere. Mannitol does not appear to worsen midline shift or precipitate neurologic decline when given as a single large bolus in humans (1.5 g/kg of body weight) (101), though mannitol does appear to draw more volume from the unaffected hemisphere (19). Although both mannitol and HS do reduce ICP and cerebral edema after ischemic stroke, robust evidence that they improve outcomes is lacking (52,102). No mention is made in the American Heart Association's scientific statement *Recommendations for the Management of Cerebral and Cerebellar Infarction With Swelling* (103).

Subarachnoid Hemorrhage

Maintaining optimal cerebral perfusion pressure (CPP) is of critical importance, especially in the context of cerebrovascular vasospasm. Bentsen and colleagues compared 7.2% HS in hydroxyethyl starch with normal saline infusions in a prospective, randomized single-blinded study. They observed a decrease in ICP as well as an improvement in CPP (104). Although no outcome information was collected, the inference is that HS may be a sound choice in this population, particularly as mannitol may have undesirable osmotic diuretic effects.

Intracerebral Hemorrhage

Similar to ischemic stroke, no mention is made of osmotherapy for cerebral edema or elevated ICP associated with ICH, which is likely due to the paucity of studies focused on this question (105). Although it may reduce ICP, regularly scheduled doses of mannitol during the first 5 days after ictus do not improve mortality or neurologic outcome vs. placebo after ICH (106) nor do they seem to change regional blood flow as detected by cranial single-photon emission computed tomography (SPECT) (107). Future dedicated clinical investigations should address the efficacy of osmotherapy in ICH.

Liver Failure

Cerebral edema may complicate fulminant hepatic failure. The mechanism of underlying cerebral edema is complex and likely multifactorial, including the alteration of cerebral hemodynamics and inflammation (108). In fact, cerebral edema may be the factor precipitating death. Both mannitol and HS have been successfully employed to alleviate cerebral edema in liver failure (109,110). However, volume status is often a challenge, particularly in cirrhosis, thus smaller volume/higher concentration osmotic agents may be warranted in such a clinical scenario.

Table 5.2 compares the different osmotic agents, their duration of action, and their adverse effects.

TABLE 5.2 Comparison of osmotherapeutic agents

	Mannitol	Hypertonic Saline	Glycerol[a]	Sorbitol[b]
Recommended Dosing	0.25–1.5 mg/kg body weight of 20% conc over 20–30 minutes	2%–7.5% as bolus or continuous infusion 30 mL of 23.4% conc over 20 minutes	Variable 10% in saline 50 grams over 1.5 or 4 hours	125 ml of 40% conc over 20 minutes
Access	Peripheral or central	Central recommended	Peripheral	Peripheral
Monitoring	Serum osmolality Calculated osmole gap	Serum sodium Serum osmolality	None	Serum glucose
Peak Effect	15–35 minutes	10–30 minutes[4]	20 minutes	20 minutes
Duration of Effect	2–4 hours	4–6 hours	1–2 hours	1–2 hours
Elimination	Renal excretion	Renal excretion	Predominantly liver	Predominantly liver
Rheologic Effect	Yes	Yes	Unknown	Unknown
Diuretic Effect	Osmotic diuretic	Diuretic action *via* ANP	Less potent osmotic diuretic	No
Hemodynamic Effect	Initial augmentation of MAP and CO. Hypotension, hypovolemia from decreased intravascular volume from diuresis.	Augments intravascular volume, maintains MAP, CVP, CO	Increases MAP, CPP, and CO	Unknown

Cellular Mechanisms	Free radical scavenger, inhibitor of apoptosis, increased oxygen delivery	Restores normal resting membrane potentials, immune modulation	Alternative source of energy, improves oxidative phosphorylation	Alternative source of energy
Potential for Rebound Edema	Yes	Potentially less than mannitol, unknown with continuous infusions	Yes, due to accumulation in cerebral tissue	Yes, due to accumulation in cerebral tissue
Adverse Effects	Hypotension, hyperkalemia, hemolysis, renal failure	Hypokalemia, congestive heart failure, hemolysis, coagulopathy, renal failure, central pontine myelinolysis (theoretical risk)	Fluid overload, hemolysis, and electrolyte disturbance. Hyperglycemia. Accumulates in brain tissue.	Hyperglycemia. Accumulates in brain tissue.

Source: Adapted with permission from. Hinson HE, Stein D, Sheth KN. Hypertonic saline and mannitol therapy in critical care neurology. *J Intensive Care Med*. 2013;28(1):3–11.

Note: MAP, mean arterial pressure; CVP, central venous pressure; CO, cardiac output; CPP, cerebral perfusion pressure; ICP, intracranial pressure; ANP, atrial natriuretic peptide.

[a]Derived from Cantore G, Guidetti B, Virno M. Oral glycerol for the reduction of intracranial pressure. *J Neurosurg*. 1964;21(4):278–283; Berger C, Sakowitz OW, Kiening KL, et al. Neurochemical monitoring of glycerol therapy in patients with ischemic brain edema. *Stroke*. 2005;36(2):e4–6.

[b]Derived from Nau R, Dreyhaupt T, Kolenda H, et al. Low blood-to-cerebrospinal fluid passage of sorbitol after intravenous infusion. *Stroke*. 1992;23(9):1276–1279.

SPECIAL CONSIDERATIONS

Renal Failure

Patients with renal insufficiency and end-stage renal disease requiring intermittent dialysis (ID) or continuous renal replacement (CRRT) are a challenge in the neurocritical care unit. These patients have a high incidence of neurological events, including idiopathic intracranial hypertension, ICH, and thromboembolic cerebrovascular events (81). Serum osmolality may be elevated due to unfiltered urea. Limited studies are available on the optimal use of osmotherapy in these patients. Mannitol is relatively contraindicated but if used should be given in the smallest effective dose possible (consider 0.5 g/kg). The use of hemodialysis to remove mannitol will expedite the half-life of the drug to 6 hours vs. 5 or more days with a GFR of less than 50 mL/min (31,82). HS may be a more effective treatment in anuric renal failure. Small studies have demonstrated the reduction of ICP and transtentorial herniation in patients with renal failure who were administered 23.4% saline (111).

Dialysis disequilibrium syndrome (DDS) leading to brain edema, herniation, and brain death has been described in neurologically injured patients undergoing CRRT and ID (112). Sodium levels for patients undergoing dialysis or CRRT must be closely monitored; as dialysate and replacement fluid is applied, serum sodium levels will trend toward 140 mEq/L (82), and more frequent redosing of HS is often needed to maintain hypernatremic goals. CRRT utilizing HS as the replacement fluid has been reported but is not routine in clinical practice (113).

Pediatric Use

The most recent recommendations for managing severe TBI in infants and children, endorsed by the American Academy of Pediatrics and the Child Neurology Society, advocated for using 3% HS to reduce intracranial hypertension rather than mannitol (114), citing insufficient evidence for the clinical use or safety of mannitol and marking a departure from their previous recommendations in 2003 (115). The authors provided level III recommendations for the use of continuous infusions of HS to maintain an ICP of less than 20 mmHg. Recommended doses of HS were 6.5 to 10 ml/kg as a bolus and 0.1 to 1.0 mL/kg of body weight per hour (114).

FUTURE DIRECTIONS

As mentioned above, few of the consensus guidelines include recommendations for the choice of osmotic agent. Practice variations in the choice of mannitol or HS, for both the dose and the administration, already exist across critical care units, which could have an impact on patient outcome (37). More clinical trials are warranted to further compare mannitol and HS and better delineate which clinical situations are more suited for one therapy vs. another.

As more research pinpoints the cellular mechanisms that cause cerebral edema, future research likely will transition from a focus on treating intracranial hypertension to inhibiting edema development. Novel therapies targeting AQP4 channels, sodium transport channels, and ATPase channels have been explored in animal models and are in the early stages of human clinical trials.

Glyburide

The sulfonylurea drug glyburide is under investigation as a potential anticytotoxic edema agent. In this context, glyburide inhibits a nonselective cation channel (sulfonylurea receptor-1 [SUR1]–regulated NC-Ca-ATP channel) expressed in the central nervous system. When activated, this channel facilitates cytotoxic edema, oncotic cell death, and vasogenic edema (116). Built on this principle and promising results in animals (117), glyburide was administered to patients in a pilot trial with large-volume (MRI lesion 82–210 cm^3) acute ischemic stroke within 10 hours of symptom onset. The incidence of malignant edema was 20%, compared to 88% in a prospective observational study of patients with driving while intoxicated (DWI) levels greater than or equal to 82 cm^3 (118). Further, eight of the 10 patients did not require osmotherapy, intubation, or decompressive hemicraniectomy (119). Based on these encouraging results, randomized placebo-controlled trials are underway in ischemic stroke (clinicaltrials.gov NCT01794182) and TBI (clinicaltrials.gov NCT01454154).

Bumetanide

Other ion channels may also play important roles in edema formation. The sodium-potassium-chloride cotransporter (NKCC1) channel regulates sodium entry into cells and is expressed into both neuronal and glial cells. Factors associated with ischemia, such as elevated levels of extracellular potassium, alterations in pH, inflammatory cytokines, and excitatory neurotransmitters such as glutamate, activate or upregulate these ion transport proteins located in the cell membrane (120,121).

Bumetanide is a FDA-approved loop diuretic and a specific inhibitor of NKCC1 at low concentrations (122). Phase I trials are currently underway to examine the efficacy of bumetanide, in addition to conventional antiepileptic medications, for the treatment of refractory neonatal seizures (clinicaltrials.gov NCT00830531). Animal studies in focal ischemia, TBI, hemorrhagic stroke, and tumors have demonstrated an attenuation of the development of cerebral edema with the administration of bumetanide (120,123,124). Human trials to evaluate its effectiveness on edema in brain-injured states, such as stroke and TBI, are forthcoming (121).

Tromethamine

Cerebral lactic acidosis, a marker of injury severity, has been linked to poor outcomes in TBI and edema formation, postulated through the regulation of pH-dependent AQP channels (125). Cerebral acidosis has also been linked to impaired glycolysis, mitochondrial dysfunction, and neuronal calcium influx (126). Although not an osmotic agent, tromethamine (THAM) is a non–CO_2-generating buffer solution that has been utilized for a variety of clinical applications, including respiratory failure, cardiac disease, liver failure, burns, diabetic ketoacidosis, renal acidosis, toxin ingestion, and malignant hyperthermia (127). THAM ameliorates brain lactic acid production and neutralizes acidosis-induced vasodilation (128). Both animal and human studies have demonstrated a reduction of ICP with infusions of THAM, as well as a reduction of edema formation and cerebral energy disturbances (128,129). A recent meta-analysis of 488 patients in 12 articles with populations being treated for different neurological conditions suggested that the use of THAM may be beneficial for reducing ICP (130) and may reduce the need for rescue osmotherapy. The exact dose and duration of therapy is unknown; most case studies administered a 0.3 molar solution of THAM as a 2 mL/kg bolus over 1 hour followed by a continuous infusion of 1 mL/kg/hr (130) for several days, targeting an arterial pH of 7.5 to 7.6. As THAM is not metabolized and is mainly excreted by the kidney, monitoring renal function is imperative. Respiratory depression from a fall in pCO_2 is common. Additional studies evaluating the timing, dosage, and prophylactic use are warranted.

CONCLUSION

Osmotic agents have proven to be a powerful tool for reducing cerebral edema and ICP for nearly half a century. In the coming decades, clinicians will likely deploy more targeted strategies to reduce edema by use of selective channel-blocking agents. Until clinical trials demonstrate the efficacy of these newer agents, mannitol and HS appear to be equally efficacious in the treatment of cerebral edema. Patient-specific considerations, such as volume status, renal function, and existing comorbidities, influence the choice of osmotherapy agents. As our understanding of the complex mechanisms underlying cerebral edema expands, future therapies will likely focus on ameliorating edema formation. Investigators must also elucidate optimal strategies for the administration (dose, timing, and format) of mannitol and HS with prospective, controlled clinical trials.

References

1. Weed LH, McKibben PS. Pressure changes in the cerebro-spinal fluid following intravenous injection of solutions of various concentrations. *Am J Physiol* [leg content]. 1919;48(4): 512–530.

2. Masserman JH. Effects of intravenous administration of hypertonic solutions of dextrose: with special reference to the cerebrospinal fluid pressure. *J Am Med Assoc*. 1934;102(25): 2084–2086.

3. Penfield W. The principles of physiology involved in the management of increased intracranial pressure. *Ann Surg*. 1935;102(4):548–554.

4. Bullock LT, Gregersen MI, Kinney R. The use of hypertonic sucrose solution intravenously to reduce cerebrospinal fluid pressure without a secondary rise. *Am J Physiol* [leg content]. 1935;112(1):82–96.

5. Hahn EV, Ramsey FB, Kohlstaedt KG. Clinical experience in the use of sucrose instead of dextrose. *J Am Med Assoc*. 1937;108(10):773–776.

6. Haden RL. Therapeutic application of the alteration of brain volume: by the intravenous injection of glucose. *J Am Med Assoc*. 1919;73(13):983–984.

7. Rigdon R, Cardwell E. Renal lesions following the intravenous injection of a hypertonic solution of sucrose: a clinical and experimental study. *Arch Intern Med*. 1942;69(4): 670–690.

8. Paczynski RP. Osmotherapy. *Crit Care Clin*. 1997;13(1):105–129.

9. Hughes J, Mudd S, Strecker EA. Reduction of increased intracranial pressure by concentrated solutions of human lyophile serum. *Arch Neurol Psychiatry*. 1938;39(6):1277 1287.

10. Javid M, Settlage P. Effect of urea on cerebrospinal fluid pressure in human subjects: preliminary report. *J Am Med Assoc*. 1956;160(11):943–949.

11. Reed DJ, Woodbury DM. Effect of hypertonic urea on cerebrospinal fluid pressure and brain volume. *J Physiol*. 1962;164(2):252–264.

12. Matson DD. Treatment of cerebral swelling. *N Engl J Med*. 1965;272(12):626–628.

13. Sweeney TE, Beuchat CA. Limitations of methods of osmometry: measuring the osmolality of biological fluids. *Am J Physiol*. 1993;264(3, pt 2):R469–480.

14. Dorwart WV, Chalmers L. Comparison of methods for calculating serum osmolality from chemical concentrations, and the prognostic value of such calculations. *Clin Chem*. 1975;21(2):190–194.

15. Oster JR, Singer I. Hyponatremia, hyposmolality, and hypotonicity: tables and fables. *Arch Intern Med*. 1999;159(4):333–336.

16. Bhagat CI, Garcia-Webb P, Fletcher E, et al. Calculated vs measured plasma osmolalities revisited. *Clin Chem*. 1984;30(10):1703–1705.

17. Badaut J, Ashwal S, Obenaus A. Aquaporins in cerebrovascular disease: a target for treatment of brain edema. *Cerebrovasc Dis*. 2011;31(6):521–531.

18. Zelenina M. Regulation of brain aquaporins. *Neurochem Int*. 2010;57(4):468–488.

19. Videen TO, Zazulia AR, Manno EM, et al. Mannitol bolus preferentially shrinks non-infarcted brain in patients with ischemic stroke. *Neurology*. 2001;57(11):2120–2122.

20. Ropper AH. Hyperosmolar therapy for raised intracranial pressure. *N Engl J Med.* 2012;367(8):746–752.

21. Ropper AH. Management of raised intracranial pressure and hyperosmolar therapy. *Pract Neurol.* 2014;14(3):152–158.

22. Gullans SR, Verbalis JG. Control of brain volume during hyperosmolar and hypoosmolar conditions. *Annu Rev Med.* 1993;44(1):289–301.

23. Lien YH, Shapiro JI, Chan L. Effects of hypernatremia on organic brain osmoles. *J Clin Invest.* 1990;85(5):1427–1435.

24. Diringer MN, Zazulia AR. Osmotic therapy. *Neurocrit Care.* 2004;1(2):219–233.

25. Wise BL, Chater N. Effect of mannitol on cerebrospinal fluid pressure: the actions of hypertonic mannitol solutions and of urea compared. *Arch Neurol.* 1961;4(2):200–202.

26. Wise BL, Chater N. The value of hypertonic mannitol solution in decreasing brain mass and lowering cerebrospinal-fluid pressure. *J Neurosurg.* 1962;19(12):1038–1043.

27. Ennis KM, Brophy GM. Management of intracranial hypertension: focus on pharmacologic strategies. *AACN Adv Crit Care.* 2011;22(3):177–182.

28. Oken DE. Renal and extrarenal considerations in high-dose mannitol therapy. *Ren Fail.* 1994;16(1):147–159.

29. García-Morales EJ, Cariappa R, Parvin CA, et al. Osmole gap in neurologic-neurosurgical intensive care unit: its normal value, calculation, and relationship with mannitol serum concentrations. *Crit Care Med.* 2004;32(4):986–991.

30. Diringer MN. New trends in hyperosmolar therapy? *Curr Opin Crit Care.* 2013;19(2): 77–82.

31. Hinson HE, Stein D, Sheth KN. Hypertonic saline and mannitol therapy in critical care neurology. *J Intensive Care Med.* 2013;28(1):3–11.

32. Alvarez B, Ferrer-Sueta G, Radi R. Slowing of peroxynitrite decomposition in the presence of mannitol and ethanol. *Free Radic Biol Med.* 1998;24(7):1331–1337.

33. Korenkov AI, Pahnke J, Frei K, et al. Treatment with nimodipine or mannitol reduces programmed cell death and infarct size following focal cerebral ischemia. *Neurosurg Rev.* 2000;23(3):145–150.

34. Suzuki J, Imaizumi S, Kayama T, et al. Chemiluminescence in hypoxic brain—the second report: cerebral protective effect of mannitol, vitamin E and glucocorticoid. *Stroke.* 1985;16(4):695–700.

35. Muizelaar JP, Lutz HA, Becker DP. Effect of mannitol on ICP and CBF and correlation with pressure autoregulation in severely head-injured patients. *J Neurosurg.* 1984;61(4): 700–706.

36. Mannitol IV Injection, Urologic Irrigation [product information]. Abraxis Pharmaceutical Products; 2006.

37. Hays AN, Lazaridis C, Neyens R, et al. Osmotherapy: Use among neurointensivists. *Neurocrit Care.* 2011;14(2):222–228.

38. Vacca VM Jr, et al. Vesicant extravasation. *Nursing.* 2014, 2013;43(9):21–22.

39. Goldwasser P, Fotino S. Acute renal failure following massive mannitol infusion appropriate response of tubuloglomerular feedback? *Arch Intern Med.* 1984;144(11):2214–2216.

40. Visweswaran P, Massin EK, Dubose TD. Mannitol-induced acute renal failure. *J Am Soc Nephrol.* 1997;8(6):1028–1033.

41. Dorman HR, Sondheimer JH, Cadnapaphornchai P. Mannitol-induced acute renal failure. *Medicine* (Baltimore). 1990;69(3):153–159.

42. Better O, Rubinstein I, Winaver J, et al. Mannitol therapy revisited (1940–1997). *Kidney Int.* 1997;52(4):886–894.

43. Coté CJ, Greenhow DE, Marshall BE. The hypotensive response to rapid intravenous administration of hypertonic solutions in man and in the rabbit. *Anesthesiology*. 1979;50(1): 30–35.

44. Domaingue CM, Nye DH. Hypotensive effect of mannitol administered rapidly. *Anaesth Intensive Care*. 1985;13(2):134–136.

45. Palma L, Bruni G, Fiaschi AI, et al. Passage of mannitol into the brain around gliomas: a potential cause of rebound phenomenon. A study on 21 patients. *J Neurosurg Sci*. 2006;50(3):63–66.

46. Sankar T, Assina R, Karis JP, et al. Neurosurgical implications of mannitol accumulation within a meningioma and its peritumoral region demonstrated by magnetic resonance spectroscopy: case report. *J Neurosurg*. 2008;108(5):1010–1013.

47. Worthley LI, Cooper DJ, Jones N. Treatment of resistant intracranial hypertension with hypertonic saline: report of two cases. *J Neurosurg*. 1988;68(3):478–481.

48. Vassar MJ, Fischer RP, O'Brien PE, et al. A multicenter trial for resuscitation of injured patients with 7.5% sodium chloride. The effect of added dextran 70. The Multicenter Group for the Study of Hypertonic Saline in Trauma Patients. *Arch Surg Chic Ill*. 1960, 1993;128(9): 1003–11;(discussion):1011–1013.

49. Berger S, Schürer L, Härtl R, et al. Reduction of post-traumatic intracranial hypertension by hypertonic/hyperoncotic saline/dextran and hypertonic mannitol. *Neurosurgery*. 1995;37(1):98–107;(discussion):107–108.

50. Mirski MA, Denchev DI, Schnitzer MS, et al. Comparison between hypertonic saline and mannitol in the reduction of elevated intracranial pressure in a rodent model of acute cerebral injury. *J Neurosurg Anesthesiol*. 2000;12(4):334–344.

51. Horn P, Münch E, Vajkoczy P, et al. Hypertonic saline solution for control of elevated intracranial pressure in patients with exhausted response to mannitol and barbiturates. *Neurol Res*. 1999;21(8):758–764.

52. Schwarz S, Georgiadis D, Aschoff A, et al. Effects of hypertonic (10%) saline in patients with raised intracranial pressure after stroke. *Stroke*. 2002;33(1):136–140.

53. Vialet R, Albanèse J, Thomachot L, et al. Isovolume hypertonic solutes (sodium chloride or mannitol) in the treatment of refractory posttraumatic intracranial hypertension: 2 mL/kg 7.5% saline is more effective than 2 mL/kg 20% mannitol. *Crit Care Med*. 2003;31(6):1683–1687.

54. Strandvik GF. Hypertonic saline in critical care: a review of the literature and guidelines for use in hypotensive states and raised intracranial pressure. *Anaesthesia*. 2009; 64(9):990–1003.

55. Ziai WC, Toung TJK, Bhardwaj A. Hypertonic saline: first-line therapy for cerebral edema? *J Neurol Sci*. 2007;261(1–2):157–166.

56. Qureshi AI, Suarez JI. Use of hypertonic saline solutions in treatment of cerebral edema and intracranial hypertension. *Crit Care Med*. 2000;28(9):3301–3313.

57. Adamides AA, Winter CD, Lewis PM, et al. Current controversies in the management of patients with severe traumatic brain injury. *ANZ J Surg*. 2006;76(3):163–174.

58. Järvelä K, Koskinen M, Kööbi T. Effects of hypertonic saline (7.5%) on extracellular fluid volumes in healthy volunteers. *Anaesthesia*. 2003;58(9):878–881.

59. Harutjunyan L, Holz C, Rieger A, et al. Efficiency of 7.2% hypertonic saline hydroxyethyl starch 200/0.5 versus mannitol 15% in the treatment of increased intracranial pressure in neurosurgical patients—a randomized clinical trial. *Crit Care*. 2005;9(5):R530–540.

60. Bhardwaj A. Osmotherapy in neurocritical care. *Curr Neurol Neurosci Rep*. 2008;7(6): 513–521.

61. Foxworthy JC, Artru AA. Cerebrospinal fluid dynamics and brain tissue composition following intravenous infusions of hypertonic saline in anesthetized rabbits. *J Neurosurg Anesthesiol.* 1990;2(4):256–265.

62. Zeng HK, Wang QS, Deng YY, et al. Hypertonic saline ameliorates cerebral edema through downregulation of aquaporin-4 expression in the astrocytes. *Neuroscience.* 2010;166(3): 878–885.

63. Cao C, Yu X, Liao Z, et al. Hypertonic saline reduces lipopolysaccharide-induced mouse brain edema through inhibiting aquaporin 4 expression. *Crit Care.* 2012;16(5):R186.

64. Thongrong C, Kong N, Govindarajan B, et al. Current purpose and practice of hypertonic saline in neurosurgery: a review of the literature. *World Neurosurg.* 2014;82(6): 1307–1318.

65. Huang L-Q, Zhu G-F, Deng Y-Y, et al. Hypertonic saline alleviates cerebral edema by inhibiting microglia-derived TNF-α and IL-1β-induced Na-K-Cl cotransporter up-regulation. *J Neuroinflammation.* 2014;11:102.

66. Elliott MB, Jallo JJ, Barbe MF, et al. Hypertonic saline attenuates tissue loss and astrocyte hypertrophy in a model of traumatic brain injury. *Brain Res.* 2009;1305:183–191.

67. Bulger EM, May S, Brasel KJ, et al. Out-of-hospital hypertonic resuscitation following severe traumatic brain injury: a randomized controlled trial. *J Am Med Assoc.* 2010;304(13): 1455–1464.

68. Ayus JC, Caputo D, Bazerque F, et al. Treatment of hyponatremic encephalopathy with a 3% sodium chloride protocol: a case series. *Am J Kidney Dis.* 2015;65(3):435–442.

69. Koenig MA, Bryan M, Lewin JL, et al. Reversal of transtentorial herniation with hypertonic saline. *Neurology.* 2008;70(13):1023–1029.

70. Qureshi AI, Suarez JI, Castro A, et al. Use of hypertonic saline/acetate infusion in treatment of cerebral edema in patients with head trauma: experience at a single center. *J Trauma.* 1999;47(4):659–665.

71. Hauer E-M, Stark D, Staykov D, et al. Early continuous hypertonic saline infusion in patients with severe cerebrovascular disease. *Crit Care Med.* 2011;39(7):1766–1772.

72. Wagner I, Hauer E-M, Staykov D, et al. Effects of continuous hypertonic saline infusion on perihemorrhagic edema evolution. *Stroke.* 2011;42(6):1540–1545.

73. Roquilly A, Mahe PJ, Latte DD, et al. Continuous controlled-infusion of hypertonic saline solution in traumatic brain-injured patients: a 9-year retrospective study. *Crit Care.* 2011;15(5):R260.

74. Sterns RH. Severe symptomatic hyponatremia: treatment and outcome. A study of 64 cases. *Ann Intern Med.* 1987;107(5):656–664.

75. Sterns RH, Cappuccio JD, Silver SM, et al. Neurologic sequelae after treatment of severe hyponatremia: a multicenter perspective. *J Am Soc Nephrol.* 1994;4(8):1522–1530.

76. Sterns RH, Riggs JE, Schochet SS. Osmotic demyelination syndrome following correction of hyponatremia. *N Engl J Med.* 1986;314(24):1535–1542.

77. Soupart A, Penninckx R, Namias B, et al. Brain myelinolysis following hypernatremia in rats. *J Neuropathol Exp Neurol.* 1996;55(1):106–113.

78. Froelich M, Ni Q, Wess C, et al. Continuous hypertonic saline therapy and the occurrence of complications in neurocritically ill patients. *Crit Care Med.* 2009;37(4): 1433–1441.

79. Qureshi AI, Suarez JI, Bhardwaj A, et al. Use of hypertonic (3%) saline/acetate infusion in the treatment of cerebral edema: effect on intracranial pressure and lateral displacement of the brain. *Crit Care Med.* 1998;26(3):440–446.

80. Prien T, Thülig B, Wüsten R, et al. Hypertonic-hyperoncotic volume replacement (7.5% NaCl/10% hydroxyethyl starch 200.000/0.5) in patients with coronary artery stenoses. *Zentralblatt Für Chir.* 1993;118(5):257–63;(discussion):264–266.

81. Brouns R, De Deyn PP. Neurological complications in renal failure: a review. *Clin Neurol Neurosurg.* 2004;107(1):1–16.

82. Kraus MA. Selection of dialysate and replacement fluids and management of electrolyte and acid-base disturbances. *Semin Dial.* 2009;22(2):137–140.

83. Lewandowski-Belfer JJ, Patel AV, Darracott RM, et al. Safety and efficacy of repeated doses of 14.6 or 23.4% hypertonic saline for refractory intracranial hypertension. *Neurocrit Care.* 2014;20(3):436–442.

84. Khanna S, Davis D, Peterson B, et al. Use of hypertonic saline in the treatment of severe refractory posttraumatic intracranial hypertension in pediatric traumatic brain injury. *Crit Care Med.* 2000;28(4):1144–1151.

85. Peterson B, Khanna S, Fisher B, et al. Prolonged hypernatremia controls elevated intracranial pressure in head-injured pediatric patients. *Crit Care Med.* 2000;28(4):1136–1143.

86. Kumar AB, Shi Y, Shotwell MS, et al. Hypernatremia is a significant risk factor for acute kidney injury after subarachnoid hemorrhage: a retrospective analysis. *Neurocrit Care.* 2015;22(2):184–191.

87. García-Sola R, Pulido P, Capilla P. The immediate and long-term effects of mannitol and glycerol. A comparative experimental study. *Acta Neurochir* (Vienna). 1991;109(3–4): 114–121.

88. Cantore G, Guidetti B, Virno M. Oral glycerol for the reduction of intracranial pressure. *J Neurosurg.* 1964;21(4):278–283.

89. Berger C, Sakowitz OW, Kiening KL, et al. Neurochemical monitoring of glycerol therapy in patients with ischemic brain edema. *Stroke.* 2005;36(2):e4–6.

90. Bardutzky J, Schwab S. Antiedema therapy in ischemic stroke. *Stroke.* 2007;38(11): 3084–3094.

91. Sloviter HA, Shimkin P, Suhara K. Glycerol as a substrate for brain metabolism. *Nature.* 1966;210(5043):1334–1336.

92. Righetti E, Celani MG, Cantisani TA, et al. Glycerol for acute stroke [online]. In: The Cochrane Collaboration, ed. *Cochrane Database of Systematic Reviews.* Chichester, UK: John Wiley and Sons, Ltd; 2004. http://doi.wiley.com/10.1002/14651858.CD000096.pub2. Accessed April 15, 2015.

93. Raslan A, Bhardwaj A. Medical management of cerebral edema. *Neurosurg Focus.* 2007;22(5):1–12.

94. Pitlick WH, Pirikitakuhlr P, Painter MJ, et al. Effects of glycerol and hyperosmolality on intracranial pressure. *Clin Pharmacol Ther.* 1982;31(4):466–471.

95. Hemmer R. Comparative studies on the drug-induced decrease in cerebral pressure. *Med Klin.* 1961;56:105–108.

96. Nau R, Dreyhaupt T, Kolenda H, et al. Low blood-to-cerebrospinal fluid passage of sorbitol after intravenous infusion. *Stroke.* 1992;23(9):1276–1279.

97. Nau R. Osmotherapy for elevated intracranial pressure: a critical reappraisal. *Clin Pharmacokinet.* 2000;38(1):23–40.

98. Rickard AC, Smith JE, Newell P, et al. Salt or sugar for your injured brain? A meta-analysis of randomised controlled trials of mannitol versus hypertonic sodium solutions to manage raised intracranial pressure in traumatic brain injury. *Emerg Med J.* 2014;31(8): 679–683.

99. Bourdeaux CP, Brown JM. Randomized controlled trial comparing the effect of 8.4% sodium bicarbonate and 5% sodium chloride on raised intracranial pressure after traumatic brain injury. *Neurocrit Care*. 2011;15(1):42–45.

100. Brain Trauma Foundation, American Association of Neurological Surgeons, Congress of Neurological Surgeons, et al. Guidelines for the management of severe traumatic brain injury. II. Hyperosmolar therapy. *J Neurotrauma*. 2007;24(suppl 1):S14–20.

101. Manno EM, Adams RE, Derdeyn CP, et al. The effects of mannitol on cerebral edema after large hemispheric cerebral infarct. *Neurology*. 1999;52(3):583–587.

102. Bereczki D, Mihálka L, Szatmári S, et al. Mannitol use in acute stroke: case fatality at 30 days and 1 year. *Stroke J Cereb Circ*. 2003;34(7):1730–1735.

103. Wijdicks EFM, Sheth KN, Carter BS, et al. Recommendations for the management of cerebral and cerebellar infarction with swelling: a statement for healthcare professionals from the American Heart Association/American Stroke Association. *Stroke*. 2014;45(4):1222–1238.

104. Bentsen G, Breivik H, Lundar T, et al. Hypertonic saline (7.2%) in 6% hydroxyethyl starch reduces intracranial pressure and improves hemodynamics in a placebo-controlled study involving stable patients with subarachnoid hemorrhage. *Crit Care Med*. 2006;34(12):2912–2917.

105. Morgenstern LB, Hemphill JC, Anderson C, et al. Guidelines for the management of spontaneous intracerebral hemorrhage: a guideline for healthcare professionals from the American Heart Association/American Stroke Association. *Stroke*. 2010;41(9):2108–2129.

106. Misra UK, Kalita J, Ranjan P, et al. Mannitol in intracerebral hemorrhage: a randomized controlled study. *J Neurol Sci*. 2005;234(1–2):41–45.

107. Kalita J, Misra UK, Ranjan P, et al. Effect of mannitol on regional cerebral blood flow in patients with intracerebral hemorrhage. *J Neurol Sci*. 2004;224(1–2):19–22.

108. Wright G, Sharifi Y, Jover-Cobos M, et al. The brain in acute on chronic liver failure. *Metab Brain Dis*. 2014;29(4):965–973.

109. Canalese J, Gimson AE, Davis C, et al. Controlled trial of dexamethasone and mannitol for the cerebral oedema of fulminant hepatic failure. *Gut*. 1982;23(7):625–629.

110. Murphy N, Auzinger G, Bernel W, et al. The effect of hypertonic sodium chloride on intracranial pressure in patients with acute liver failure. *Hepatol Baltim Md*. 2004;39(2):464–470.

111. Hirsch KG, Spock T, Koenig MA, et al. Treatment of elevated intracranial pressure with hyperosmolar therapy in patients with renal failure. *Neurocrit Care*. 2012;17(3):388–394.

112. Osgood M, Compton R, Carandang R, et al. Rapid unexpected brain herniation in association with renal replacement therapy in acute brain injury: caution in the neurocritical care unit. *Neurocrit Care*. 2015;22(2):176–183.

113. Rifkin SI, Malek AR, Behrouz R. Use of hypertonic continuous venovenous hemodiafiltration to control intracranial hypertension in an end-stage renal disease patient. SAGE-Hindawi Access to *Research Int J of Nephrol*. Volume 2010, Article ID 391656, 2 pages. doi:10.4061/2010/391656.

114. Kochanek PM, Carney N, Adelson PD, et al. Guidelines for the acute medical management of severe traumatic brain injury in infants, children, and adolescents—second edition. *Pediatr Crit Care Med*. 2012;13(suppl 1):S1–82.

115. Adelson PD, Bratton SL, Carney NA, et al. Guidelines for the acute medical management of severe traumatic brain injury in infants, children, and adolescents. Chapter 11. Use of hyperosmolar therapy in the management of severe pediatric traumatic brain injury. *Pediatr Crit Care Med*. 2003;4(suppl 3):S40–44.

116. Simard JM, Tarasov KV, Gerzanich V. Non-selective cation channels, transient receptor potential channels and ischemic stroke. *Biochim Biophys Acta*. 2007;1772(8):947–957.

117. Simard JM, Yurovsky V, Tsymbalyuk N, et al. Protective effect of delayed treatment with low-dose glibenclamide in three models of ischemic stroke. *Stroke J Cereb Circ.* 2009;40(2): 604–609.

118. Thomalla G, Hartmann F, Juettler E, et al. Prediction of malignant middle cerebral artery infarction by magnetic resonance imaging within 6 hours of symptom onset: a prospective multicenter observational study. *Ann Neurol.* 2010;68(4):435–445.

119. Sheth KN, Kimberly WT, Elm JJ, et al. Pilot study of intravenous glyburide in patients with a large ischemic stroke. *Stroke J Cereb Circ.* 2014;45(1):281–283.

120. Song D, Xu J, Du T, et al. Inhibition of brain swelling after ischemia-reperfusion by β-adrenergic antagonists: correlation with increased K^+ and decreased Ca^{2+} concentrations in extracellular fluid. *BioMed Res Int.* 2014;2014:1–10.

121. Walcott BP, Kahle KT, Simard JM. Novel treatment targets for cerebral edema. *Neurotherapeutics.* 2012;9(1):65–72.

122. Staley KJ. Wrong-way chloride transport: is it a treatable cause of some intractable seizures? *Epilepsy Curr.* 2006;6(4):124–127.

123. Wang G, Huang H, He Y, et al. Bumetanide protects focal cerebral ischemia-reperfusion injury in rat. *Int J Clin Exp Pathol.* 2014;7(4):1487.

124. Lu K-T, Cheng N-C, Wu C-Y, et al. NKCC1-mediated traumatic brain injury-induced brain edema and neuron death via Raf/MEK/MAPK cascade. *Crit Care Med.* 2008;36(3): 917–922.

125. Tran ND, Kim S, Vincent HK, et al. Aquaporin-1–mediated cerebral edema following traumatic brain injury: effects of acidosis and corticosteroid administration. *J Neurosurg.* 2009; 112(5):1095–1104.

126. Goldman SA, Pulsinelli WA, Clarke WY, et al. The effects of extracellular acidosis on neurons and glia in vitro. *J Cereb Blood Flow Metab.* 1989;9(4):471.

127. Nahas GG, Sutin KM, Fermon C, et al. Guidelines for the treatment of acidaemia with THAM. *Drugs.* 1998;55(2):191–224.

128. Wolf AL, Levi L, Marmarou A, et al. Effect of THAM upon outcome in severe head injury: a randomized prospective clinical trial. *J Neurosurg.* 1993;78(1):54–59.

129. Zeiler FA, Gillman LM, Teitelbaum J, et al. Early implementation of THAM for ICP control: therapeutic hypothermia avoidance and reduction in hypertonics/hyperosmotics [online]. In: *Case Rep Crit Care;* Volume 2014 (2014), Article ID 139342, 4 pages.

130. Zeiler FA, Teitelbaum J, Gillman LM, et al. THAM for control of ICP. *Neurocrit Care.* 2014;21(2):332–344.

6

Metabolic Suppression and Induced Hypothermia for the Treatment of Intracranial Hypertension

Chad M. Miller

INTRODUCTION

Metabolic suppression and targeted temperature management (TTM) are fundamental strategies utilized in the tiered approach to either sudden or refractory intracranial hypertension (IH). The application of each denotes the diagnosis of a critical clinical state and necessitates a sound understanding of the benefits, risks, and options inherent with either approach. This chapter will explore these treatment modalities independently and address the pathophysiology, clinical efficacy, and practical treatment pearls relevant to both.

METABOLIC SUPPRESSION AND INTRACRANIAL PRESSURE CONTROL

Metabolic suppression is a commonly used approach to both acute intracranial pressure (ICP) spikes and prolonged refractory IH due to diffuse or focal sources. Metabolic suppression can be accomplished with the use of opioids, benzodiazepines, barbiturates, alpha receptor agonists, and other sedative hypnotics. Because of the diverse characteristics of medications used to achieve metabolic suppression, great versatility exists regarding the timing and intensiveness of its role.

The Pathophysiology of Metabolic Suppression in Intracranial Hypertension

Despite recent debate regarding the value of ICP-directed treatments, strong data exist correlating the elevation of ICP with negative outcomes. This has been shown in subarachnoid hemorrhage (SAH), traumatic brain injury (TBI), brain tumors, and a host of other pathologies (1,2). The Monro-Kellie doctrine states that ICP is dictated by the volume of the contents of the rigid cranial vault (3). Changes in the volume of the cerebrospinal fluid (CSF) and blood represent not only pathologies but also opportunities to treat elevated pressures. For the patient with intact cerebral autoregulation, cerebral blood flow (CBF), and therefore blood volume, directly depends upon the metabolic needs of the brain (4). Cerebral requirements vary substantially, and arousal levels, cognitive function, fever, and pathology all influence them. It has been postulated that 50% of the brain's metabolic activity is essential to maintain cellular structural integrity. The balance of energy is directed toward generating and conducting neuronal electrical activity (5) and is thus eligible for temporary suppression to minimize cranial blood volume. For patients with intact coupling of metabolism and CBF, the reduction of ICP using sedative agents occurs chiefly by this mechanism.

Shivering, body tremors, motor agitation, and dyssynchrony with the mechanical ventilator may also cause elevations in ICP. The use of sedative agents may benefit ICP control by mitigating these noncerebral irritants.

Other postulated means for sedative control of IH include free radical scavenging, increased vascular resistance, and the reduction of systemic CO_2 production (2). Lower systemic CO_2 causes vasoconstriction of capacitance vasculature and may represent the chief reason for ICP reduction when coupling is not preserved (6).

Support for Clinical Efficacy

The efficacy of pharmaceutical metabolic suppression for treating IH can be assessed in multiple ways. Widespread evidence exists to support the ICP-lowering effects of treatment (7–11). However, demonstrations of improvement in short- and long-term clinical outcomes have been more elusive. Although light sedation is often used to help with patient agitation, deep sedative therapy for ICP management is often implemented only after hyperosmolar therapy, CO_2 modulation, surgery, paralysis, CSF drainage, and head positioning have failed to achieve control. As a result, a historical failure to demonstrate the clinical benefit of metabolic suppression may result from an unmodifiable trajectory of decline characteristic of this patient cohort. This is certainly the case in prior studies of pentobarbital, in which dosing has been generally reserved for salvage therapy or as a third-tier or fourth-tier measure (12). Furthermore, many agents rely upon CBF-metabolic coupling as the chief mechanism for IH control. This coupling is not maintained late in the course of elevated ICP at the time that metabolic suppression is employed. Likewise, the most seriously brain-injured patients often possess severe systemic injury. The correlations of systemic injury with recovery confound outcome measures based upon patient recovery.

One meta-analysis of pentobarbital use in severe TBI patients saw no benefit in IH improvement (13). Despite this, pentobarbital infusions have been shown to increase brain oxygen content ($PbtO_2$) independent of their effects on ICP lowering (2). However, when used late and with poorly controlled IH, the use of pentobarbital can be deleterious to brain oxygenation. These associations are often difficult to decipher given the numerous factors regulating cerebral oxygenation (FiO_2, $PaCO_2$, etc.).

Propofol is novel in that it does not impair cerebral autoregulation at high doses (6). It is also a favored agent given its rapid onset and short duration of action. In one series of severe TBI patients titrated to a propofol electroencephalogram (EEG) suppression of 4 to 8 seconds, mean ICP fell from 20 ± 10 mmHg to 16 ± 11 mmHg ($P < 0.001$). In these same patients, CBF was reduced by $16 \pm 11\%$ ($p < 0.001$), and jugular bulb saturations increased (72 ± 8 to $75 \pm 8\%$, $p = 0.003$). This same study concluded that metabolic suppression with propofol was superior to induced hypertension in regard to ICP reduction (6). A high CBF prior to suppression predicted the effectiveness of ICP control.

Therapeutic Targets for Metabolic Suppression

EEG has been the gold standard for monitoring the depth of sedation and its impact on CBF (5). As the brain is sedated, the EEG proceeds through a progression of electrical changes. Initially, beta activity is seen with clinical amnesia and anxiolysis. Deeper sedation results in delta and theta activity with deeper stages of unconsciousness and coma, ultimately correlating with suppression of the electrical waveform (5) (see Figure 6.1). Although these responses are predictable and reproducible between patients, a target titration to achieve the maximal benefit of metabolic suppression remains a controversial topic. Cortical EEG is not reflective of deep structure metabolism, which may comprise 40% to 50% of the metabolic activity in an awake patient (14).

Previous conventional wisdom deduced that a maximal ICP-lowering effect could be consistently correlated with a suppression duration of around 20

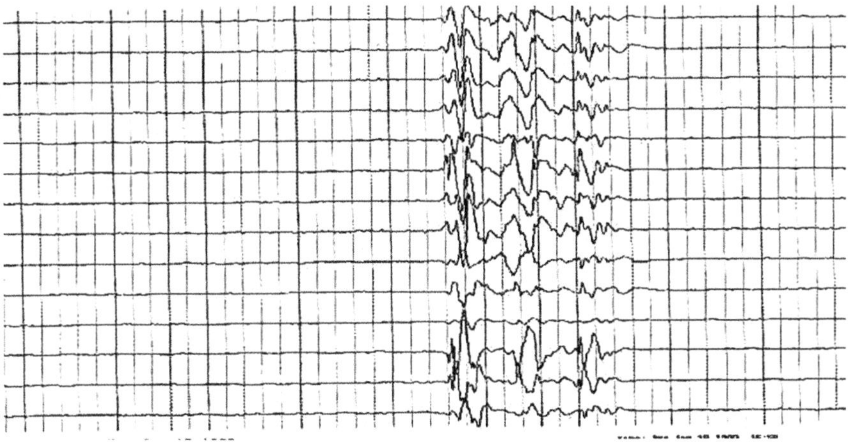

FIGURE 6.1 Suppressed electroencephalogram with transient burst pattern seen in a patient receiving sedative agents for the purpose of intracranial pressure control.

seconds (15). However, in a small case of surgical patients undergoing metabolic suppression, it was shown that electrical flatlining might result in a further reduction of CBF (14). Therefore, burst suppression may not be optimal. Further confounding this issue is the notion that other pathophysiologic means, such as neuroprotection, might represent a more appropriate titration goal than CBF lowering. ICP represents only a single pathway of potential secondary injury. Since many suppressing medications are thought to minimize injury through an assortment of methods, perhaps multimodal neuromonitoring parameters should be utilized to guide metabolic suppression (2).

The interpretive expertise required to manage this continuous monitor limits EEG. As a result, substantial interest has arisen regarding the use of more objective monitoring devices that can be nursing directed. Bispectral index (BIS) technology may be simpler to analyze and has been associated with lower monitoring costs (5). BIS is a global monitor, originally designed to assess responses to sedation and anesthesia in the operative environment. It acquires EEG from a frontal-temporal montage, which is converted to a linear scale ranging from 0 to 100 (5). A value of 0 corresponds to minimal to no brain activity, while 100 is consistent with an awake state. A suppression rate (BIS SR) can also be calculated that describes the number of EEG bursts in the previous 63-second interval. As a derived EEG parameter, strong correlations have been reported between EEG burst rate and BIS SR and BIS value (16). In one study, the inverse Spearman rank coefficient between EEG burst count and

BIS SR showed excellent correlation (SR coefficient=−0.8727) (5). Obviously, what BIS might gain in simplicity is offset by its lack of specificity. Many of these patients remain at high risk for subclinical seizures, and there is great value in the type of data derived from conventional EEG. No numeric BIS targets have been validated for use in guiding the metabolic suppression of IH.

Patients with IH resulting from multilesional intracranial injury can have prolonged and unpredictable durations of elevated ICP. Despite this knowledge, it is unclear how metabolic suppression should be weaned following the resolution of IH. It would be prudent to continue brain monitoring throughout the extent of sedative weaning and for a duration of time thereafter. The rate of weaning should likewise be slow and consider the unique pace of drug clearance for each patient.

Risks and Comparison of Suppression Agents

Few comparisons exist regarding any metric of efficacy for the commonly used suppression agents. The choice of drug often depends upon its side-effect profile and other sedation needs.

Propofol is a lipid-soluble hypnotic/amnestic agent popular for its quick onset, clearance, and easy titration. It has the benefit of not disrupting flow metabolism coupling and may have antioxidant properties capable of limiting secondary brain injury (14). Propofol can be a cardiac depressant and result in significant hypotension. Prolonged use can also place the patient at risk for propofol infusion syndrome, a potentially lethal dose-related phenomenon marked by hepatic dysfunction, elevated creatine kinase levels, hypertriglyceridemia, and acidosis (17). Dosing approaching 100 mcg/kg/min intravenous (IV) continuous infusion may be required to achieve the desired suppression in many patients.

Barbiturates are a common class of medications utilized for metabolic suppression. Thiopental is often used in the operative setting, particularly for neurosurgical procedures. Pentobarbital is frequently used in the critical care setting, and dosages of 0.3 to 7.5 mg/kg/hr have been shown to be effective in suppressing burst activity (2). Despite being effective suppressants, barbiturates have a side-effect profile that includes hypotension, immunosuppression, hepatotoxicity, and arrhythmias. Additionally, pentobarbital is a smooth muscle relaxant that may result in gastroparesis or lobar lung collapse due to laxity of the musculature in the distributing airways (18). Cerebral autoregulation is typically disrupted at higher dosing ranges. As a result, persistent IH in the setting of metabolic suppression should prompt an assessment for excessive perfusing pressure resulting in sustained elevations in ICP (Figure 6.2).

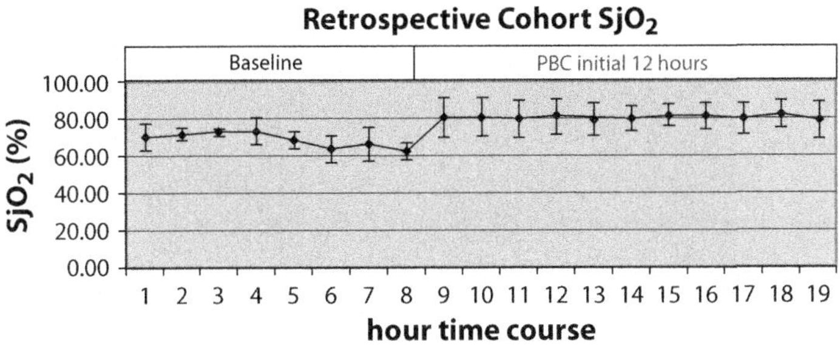

FIGURE 6.2 Retrospective cohort SjO_2. Impact of metabolic suppression with pentobarbital on mean jugular venous bulb oxygen saturation. Metabolic suppression correlates with elevation in oxygen saturation and hyperemia in a subset of patients. Hyperemia may explain inadequate intracranial pressure (ICP) control despite successful metabolic suppression. *Note:* PBC, pentobarbital coma.

Benzodiazepines are popular agents used to achieve metabolic suppression. Midazolam, perhaps the most commonly used agent, requires doses substantially higher than those used for other indications to achieve electrographic suppression. Fatty tissues in the body can store midazolam, resulting in an effective drug half-life much longer than expected based upon serological clearance. Metabolic acidosis can result from infusion of the solvent propylene glycol, which can complicate the use of high-dose continuous lorazepam infusions. In one study, nearly half of all patient samples showed complications related to accumulation during lorazepam use (19).

Other medications, such as ketamine and dexmedetomidine, have been used anecdotally for the purpose of metabolic suppression. Dexmedetomidine is unique in that it does not cause significant respiratory depression. The clinical value of these medications is unknown, and both require further study regarding their role in IH control.

Opioid medications, such as morphine, hydromorphone, and fentanyl, do not likely play a role in long-term use for metabolic suppression. In the setting of acute ICP elevation, bolus doses may be given in combination with other sedative medications to try to gain immediate control of IH. Hypotension and gastroparesis often complicate chronic use (20).

TARGETED TEMPERATURE MANAGEMENT AND INTRACRANIAL PRESSURE CONTROL

The impact of temperature upon metabolic rate and ICP has long been recognized. In recent years, interest has increased in utilizing temperature control to lessen secondary injury, control metabolism, and optimize cerebral perfusion throughout a variety of neurological diagnoses (21). The appeal of this approach arises from the broad, sweeping physiologic impact of fever management and induced cooling.

The Pathophysiologic Benefits of Targeted Temperature Management for the Control of Intracranial Pressure

Two distinct rationales exist for the consideration of TTM after brain injury: the control of ICP through the alteration of cerebral metabolism and neuroprotection. Although this chapter focuses upon the role of TTM for the specific purpose of ICP control, the two benefits of temperature modulation are tightly interrelated and must be collectively considered.

Most cellular biochemical processes are temperature dependent (7). The number and complexity of these physiologic pathways varies with the type and nature of the initial neurological insult. For instance, the purely ischemic injury of thrombotic stroke stands in relative contrast to the compressive, ischemic, and hemorrhagic nature of TBI. Accordingly, the potential impact of neuroprotection should be expected to be inconsistent between patient and injury type. The possible physiologic benefits of TTM include reduced edema formation and inflammatory mediators, mitigation of reperfusion, reduced blood–brain barrier permeability, and suppression of epileptic activity (7,22). Furthermore, temperature management similarly alters free radical production, apoptosis, oxidative stress, and mitochondrial function. In animal models of ischemia, mild hypothermia has been shown to reduce perilesional elevations of glutamate, which is a mediator of edema and inflammation (23). Hypothermia has also been shown to reduce posttraumatic levels of aspartate, hydroxyl radicals, and cytokine production by microglia (24). An elevation in inflammatory cytokines after brain trauma correlates with worsened clinical outcome (23). Contrary to the host of unsuccessful neuroprotective agents designed to target a specific pathway of secondary injury, TTM remains an intriguing therapeutic approach due to its mechanistic multiplicity.

Like sedative-mediated suppression, TTM may also exhibit ICP-lowering effects through metabolic alteration. Fever has been shown to increase cerebral metabolic rates by 10% to 13% per Celsius degree of elevation (24). Furthermore, brain metabolism is reduced by 5% to 7% for every Celsius degree that cooling achieves (25). In brain regions near posttraumatic contusions, hypothermia reduces anaerobic glycolysis and lactate to pyruvate ratios (26). The consequence of each of these findings is a lowering of the requisite CBF. In animal models of cooling for ICP control, CBF reductions were seen to correlate with the depth of cooling (29°C = 77% reduction vs. 33°C = 56% reduction) (23). There may be limits to this benefit, however. Interestingly, CBF and $CMRO_2$ become uncoupled at lower temperatures and are associated with evidence of ischemic injury (23,27). Some studies have shown that hypothermia preferentially reduces functional metabolism but not basal metabolic rate (28). This specificity is potentially beneficial and would explain why the impact of hypothermia upon CBF is variable throughout multiple trials, considering the disparate metabolic states of the individual subjects (29).

In summary, the ICP-lowering effects of TTM have the potential to be more robust than that achieved with sedative-induced metabolic suppression since cooling possesses potential neuroprotective properties. Obviously, even rapid cooling lacks the capacity to respond to emergent critical IH, thus limiting this approach to ongoing refractory ICP elevation.

Support for the Clinical Efficacy of Targeted Temperature Management With Intracranial Pressure Lowering

Enthusiasm for TTM in patients with IH arises from benefits in outcome observed for patients experiencing cardiac arrest and perinatal asphyxia (30–34). The value of cooling that these patients realize likely derives from neuroprotection as opposed to ICP control. However, a reduction of cerebral edema and death has been shown in animal studies exploring TTM for purposes of ICP management (35–38). Refractory ICP is most prevalent among those patients with traumatic brain insults, which account for over 50,000 deaths annually in the United States (39). As a result, the merit of TTM has been most fully explored in patients with TBI.

A review by Polderman noted significant improvement in ICP in 17 controlled trials of TTM for TBI patients with ICP elevations refractory to standard medical treatment (7). Many other single-center trials and case series corroborated these findings, and the majority demonstrated short-term benefits in outcome attributable to cooling (40). Improvements in outcome were seen despite the inconsistent implementation of TTM, slow cooling, and the inexperienced management of TTM side effects (7). This promise led to the launch of a multicenter trial of 392 severe TBI patients who were randomized to standard medical management or cooling to 33°C for 48 hours. The cooled cohort did not realize the study end point of an improved 6-month functional outcome (41). Given the wealth of preceding data to support the benefits of cooling, the results of this study were surprising and ascribed to intercenter variance in outcomes and low body temperatures in the control groups. The series of published trials revealed several lessons regarding the use of TTM in severe

TBI patients. The duration of cooling, type of brain trauma, subject inclusion criteria, and rewarming rates tended to have a significant impact upon successful patient management. Nonetheless, the efficacy of TTM after TBI with regard to an improved outcome is still unproven in a multicenter controlled trial. Although the trial consistently demonstrated improvement in ICP with cooling, this was a secondary end point in each of the trials. The Eurotherm 3235 trial intends to prospectively assess the benefit of TTM for ICP control as a primary measure in 600 severe TBI patients (42).

TTM has been explored for ICP control in other diagnostic groups. Reductions in ICP have been demonstrated in aneurysmal subarachnoid hemorrhage (aSAH) patients (43). Anecdotal evidence suggests that cooling may serve as an advantageous bridge for ICP control peri–liver transplantation. Temperature reduction not only tempers diffuse edema but may have added benefit in modulating ammonia metabolism (44). In a cohort of 13 patients with hepatic failure, mean ICP was reduced from 36.5 to 16.3 mmHg with cooling to 32°C to 33°C (45). The exploration of TTM after ischemic stroke has focused more on reducing ischemia than treating IH. Nonetheless, improvements in stroke survival have been suggested after TTM, despite post-rewarming ICP rebounding (46).

A review of the current data for TTM after acute brain injury reveals overwhelming evidence in favor of its benefits for ICP lowering but a paucity of findings demonstrating improved clinical outcomes. ICP treatments, historically, have not been held to the standard of whether they improve outcome but rather that they control ICP. Given the complexity of factors affecting outcomes and survival in these patients, it is debatable which end point is more appropriate. In assessing treatments for ICP control, one review found hypothermia to be at least as effective as hyperventilation, mannitol, and barbiturates but perhaps less effective than hypertonic saline, lumbar CSF drainage, and decompressive hemicraniectomy (22).

Clinical Targeted Temperature Management Goals

Though perhaps not any more proven than induced hypothermia, avoiding fever has become a mainstay of clinical practice in the neurocritical care unit. The adverse impact of fever upon outcome is well recognized and has been reported for ischemic stroke, intracerebral hemorrhage (ICH), aSAH, and TBI (47–50). The potential benefit of targeted normothermia may be more relevant to neuroprotection than ICP control, but benefits likely exist for both therapeutic goals (51). After ischemic stroke, the risk of an adverse outcome increases 2.2% for every Celsius degree increase in temperature (52). Similar findings are reported for ICH and aSAH (53–54). Metabolic disturbance is common with mild temperature elevations and may be reduced through TTM (55) (see Figure 6.3). A historically controlled trial of normothermia after TBI demonstrated improved ICP management simply by using an indwelling cooling catheter that maintained tighter fever control (56). Given the relative safety of normothermia maintenance and the established consequence of fever to the

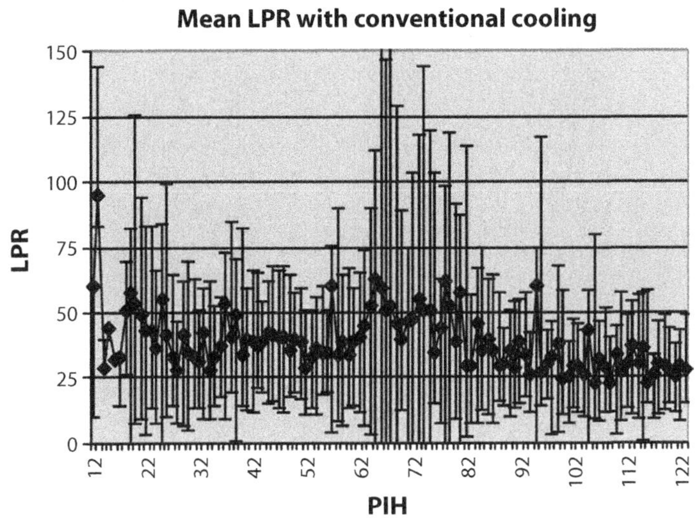

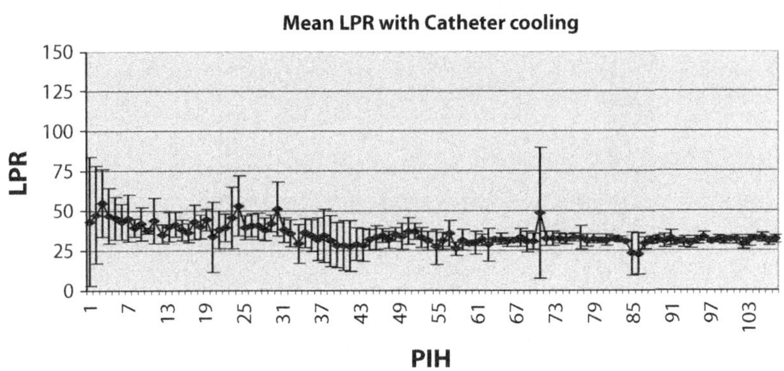

FIGURE 6.3 Mean lactate to pyruvate ratio (LPR) with conventional cooling (upper graph) and mean LPR with catheter cooling (lower graph). Graphs showing LPR among patients undergoing conventional (2A) and catheter-directed (2B) normothermia after traumatic brain injury. Improved mean temperature control and less metabolic distress is seen in those treated with intravascular cooling. *Note:* PIH, post-injury hour

injured brain, it is unlikely normothermia will bear the same burden of proof for therapeutic benefit that is sought for induced hypothermia.

Defined risks exist when inducing mild hypothermia, and achieving a margin of therapeutic benefit is contingent upon appropriately monitoring and implementing TTM. Body temperature should be measured in a manner that best approximates the true temperature of the brain. Difference in temperatures between the brain and body exist and can approach two full Celsius degrees in the febrile state (51). When available, actual brain temperature acquired through an implanted probe should be used for directing therapy. Preferred alternatives include intravascular temperature acquired through a pulmonary artery catheter or rectal, bladder, or esophageal probes. Surface, oral, or axillary temperature are insufficient and tend to deviate greatly from internal temperatures during surface vasoconstriction.

Several commercial devices are available to assist in the induction, maintenance, and rewarming phases of TTM. These achieve cooling either through circulating chilled water through adhesive skin wraps or perfusing chilled saline through closed-circuit intravascular catheters. When compared, these two methods have comparable efficacy and time to target temperatures (57). One study suggests that temperatures very less with intravascular catheters. Regardless of the technique chosen, utilizing a cooling strategy with real-time, direct-temperature feedback regulation is valuable in avoiding temperature overshoot and reducing the nursing effort required for cooling. Useful reviews are available that provide detailed guidance for TTM (58).

Limited data is available regarding the most appropriate temperature target for ICP control. Goals of 32°C to 34°C are often considered safe, though temperatures throughout the mild hypothermia range have not been extensively compared (59). One small report suggested that cooling below 35°C may not confer additional benefit for ICP reduction (60). To date, most goals are chosen with the intent to minimize cooling-related side effects.

The beneficial duration of cooling is likely specific to the patient and disease type. Retrospective reviews of TTM for ICP-lowering trials in TBI patients suggest that an extended length of cooling may be associated with improved outcomes (61). Unfortunately, a prolonged duration of cooling also increases the risk of TTM-related side effects. If cooling is required for refractory IH, there is great likelihood that the duration of treatment must meet or exceed 48 to 72 hours. Furthermore, in multiple trials, rebound IH was seen with rapid weaning of hypothermia for ICP reduction (40,41). Slow rewarming at rates of 0.25°C per hour are likely needed to avoid this complication.

The Risk of Targeted Temperature Management for Intracranial Pressure Reduction

An attentive and protocolized approach to TTM is necessary to minimize cooling risks (58). Targeting and maintaining a cooling range deemed safe (T = 32°C–35°C) can also mitigate many risks (7). Cooling below 30°C has been associated with exceptional risks, including disordered coagulation, dysrhythmias, and impaired liver function (62).

The most significant risk complicating TTM is body shivering. Shivering can exacerbate IH and increase metabolic expenditure (63). Shivering depletes adenosine triphosphate (ATP) stores within the body, often in individuals already suffering from a hypermetabolic state (64). The first and most important step in limiting shivering is having an established process for its recognition and quantification. The Bedside Shivering Assessment Score (BSAS) is a 4-point scale that is among the most utilized measures for tracking cooling-related shivering (63) (see Figure 6.4). A tiered and automated approach to shiver management should be outlined in an established treatment protocol and order set (58,63). Effective strategies to minimize shivering include surface counterwarming, meperidine, magnesium, buspirone, narcotics, paralytics, and dexmedetomidine.

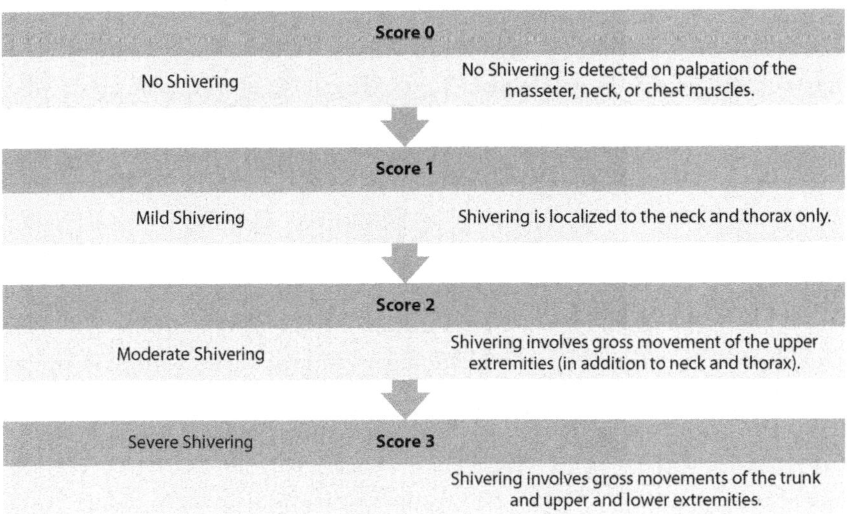

FIGURE 6.4 Bedside Shivering Assessment Score (BSAS). The BSAS is a 4-point scale that allows an objective assessment of the degree of shivering to guide therapy (14).

Numerous other risks accompany the implementation of TTM. Ten percent of hypothermic subjects in Clifton's TBI trial experienced hypotension (65). Bradycardia and cold diuresis may aggravate this complication (66). Other common risks include decreased insulin secretion, increased sympathetic discharge, pulmonary infections, hypokalemia, and thrombocytopenia (66). Hypothermia reduces the rate of clearance of cytochrome P450–metabolized medications by 7% to 22% for every Celsius degree of lowering (67). Prolonged cooling may result in complications due to impairment of the host inflammatory response (22). The cardiac arrest literature has revealed that short-term mild cooling is extremely safe when appropriately employed. The extended durations of treatment required for IH may result in greater rates of cooling-associated risks.

A COMPARISON OF TARGETED TEMPERATURE MANAGEMENT AND SEDATIVE METABOLIC SUPPRESSION

Both TTM and sedative metabolic suppression are powerful tools useful in the treatment of refractory IH. The relative benefits of the two therapies have not been systemically compared. Both utilize a reduction of cerebral metabolism because of its primary influence on CBF requirements. Despite this similarity, the portion of metabolism affected may differ between the two strategies. Hypothermia appears to delay neuronal membrane depolarization longer than sedative therapy, despite a comparable impact on $CMRO_2$. As a result TTM may confer benefits in regard to ATP depletion, neuroprotection, and the preservation of neuronal structural integrity (68). These concepts remain theoretical at present and superior clinical outcomes have not yet validated them.

CHOOSING THE CORRECT END POINT: IS INTRACRANIAL PRESSURE OUR BEST (AND ONLY) TARGET?

This chapter has focused upon achieving conventionally regarded ICPs in the acute injured brain. This discussion deserves the caveat that ICP control alone may not be an acceptable therapeutic target. Recently, the Benchmark Evidence from South American Trials: Treatment of Intracranial Pressure (BEST TRIPS) trial reported that an ICP-directed treatment paradigm failed to reduce mortality compared to a radiologic guided algorithm (69). Criticism exists regarding the legitimacy of the protocols studied and the applicability of the clinical environment to modern neurocritical care practice. Nonetheless, an appropriate analysis of the study shows that care predicated exclusively upon ICP management is likely to yield unacceptable outcomes. Accounting for the various mechanisms by which metabolic suppression and TTM have an impact on brain function, one must consider whether a more expansive consideration of the brain's needs should guide thresholds for therapy. The continuous monitoring of brain oxygenation, blood flow, and metabolism may reveal more suitable clinical goals.

Likewise, the Lund strategy of acute brain injury management deemphasizes the role of ICP (70). Lund fundamental concepts include a prioritization of CBF over ICP, the maintenance of intracapillary hydrostatic pressure, a liberal use of sedation, and targeted vasoconstriction. Although evidence for the benefits of this approach are limited, multiple studies have shown that secondary injury is often prevalent despite an adherence to ICP and cerebral perfusion pressure treatment thresholds (71–73).

CONCLUSION

TTM and metabolic suppression play an important role in the management of the acutely and critically brain-injured patient. The complexity and diversity of patients suffering from IH have limited our understanding of the appropriate targets and value associated with these therapies. This chapter provides a reasonable clinical reference based upon available data. Further research is needed to clarify their efficacy and widen the margins between therapeutic risks and benefits.

References

1. Perez-Barcena J, Barcelo B, Homar J, et al. Comparison of the effectiveness of pentobarbital and thiopental in patients with refractory intracranial hypertension. *Neurocirugia.* 2005;16:5–13.

2. Chen HI, Malhotra N, Oddo M, et al. Barbiturate infusion for intractable intracranial hypertension and its effect on brain oxygenation. *Neurosurg.* 2008;63:880–887.

3. Schaller B, Graf R. Different compartments of intracranial pressure and its relationship to cerebral blood flow. *J Trauma.* 2005;59(6):1521–1531.

4. Czonyka M, Miller C. Monitoring of cerebral autoregulation. *Neurocrit Care.* 2014; (suppl 2):S95–102.

5. Arbour RB, Dissin J. Predictive value of the bispectral index for burst suppression on diagnostic electroencephalogram during drug-induced coma. *J of Neuroscience Nurs.* 2015;47(2): 113–122.

6. Oertel M, Kelly DF, Lee JH, et al. Efficacy of hyperventilation, blood pressure elevation, and metabolic suppression therapy in controlling intracranial pressure after head injury. *J Neurosurg.* 2002;97:1045–1053.

7. Polderman KH. Induced hypothermia and fever control for prevention and treatment of neurological injuries. *Lancet*. 2008;371:1955–1969.

8. Harbaugh RD, James HE, Marshall LF, et al. Acute therapeutic modalities for experimental vasogenic edema. *Neurosurg*. 1979;5:656–665.

9. Hoff JT, Marshall L. Barbiturates in neurosurgery. *Clin Neurosurg*. 1979;637–642.

10. Marshall LF, Smith RW, Shapiro HM. The outcome with aggressive treatment in severe head injuries. Part II: acute and chronic barbiturate administration in the management of head injury. *J Neurosurg*. 1979;50:26–30.

11. Rea GL, Rockswold GL. Barbiturate therapy in uncontrolled intracranial hypertension. *Neurosurg*. 1983;12:401–404.

12. Stevens RD, Huff JS, Duckworth J, et al. Emergency neurological life support: intracranial hypertension and herniation. *Neurocrit Care*. 2012;(suppl 1):S60–65.

13. Roberts I. Barbiturates for acute traumatic brain injury. *Cochrane Database Syst Rev*. 2000;136:CD000033.

14. Doyle PW, Matta BF. Burst suppression or isoelectric encephalogram for cerebral protection: evidence from metabolic suppression studies. *British J of Anes*. 1999;83(4):580–584.

15. Venkatapura R, Rao U, Ganne S. Quantification of burst suppression and bispectral index with 2 different bolus doses of thiopentone sodium. *J of Neurosurg Anes*. 2007;19(3): 179–182.

16. Riker RR, Fraser GL, Wilkens ML. Comparing the bispectral index and suppression ratio with burst suppression of the electroencephalogram during pentobarbital infusions in adult intensive care patients. *Pharmacotherapy*. 2003;23(9):1087–1093.

17. Pisapia JM, Wendell LC, Kumar MA, et al. Lactate to pyruvate ratio as a marker of propofol infusion syndrome after subarachnoid hemorrhage. *Neurocrit Care*. 2011;15(1): 134–138.

18. Sadaka F, Veremakis C. Therapeutic hypothermia for the management of intracranial hypertension in severe traumatic brain injury: a systematic review. *Brain Injury*. 2012;26(7–8): 899–908.

19. Horinek EL, Kiser TH, Fish DN, et al. Propylene glycol accumulation in critically ill patients receiving continuous intravenous lorazepam infusions. *Ann Pharmacother*. 2009;43(12): 1964–1671.

20. Memis D, Inal MT, Kavalci G, et al. Intravenous paracetamol reduced the use of opioids, extubation time, and opioid-related adverse effects after major surgery in intensive care unit. *J Crit Care*. 2010;25(3):458–462.

21. Perman DM, Goyal M, Neumar RW, et al. Clinical applications of targeted temperature management. *Chest*. 2014;145(2):386–393.

22. Schreskinger M, Marion DW. Contemporary management of traumatic intracranial hypertension: is there a role for therapeutic hypothermia? *Neurocrit Care*. 2009;11:427–436.

23. Mori M, Maeda M, Miyazaki M, et al. Effects of mild (33 degrees C) and moderate (29 degrees C) hypothermia on cerebral blood flow and metabolism, lactate, and extracellular glutamate in experimental head injury. *Neural Res*. 1998;20(8):719–726.

24. Rangel-Castillo L, Robertson CS. Management of intracranial hypertension [abstract ix]. *Crit Care Clin*. 2006;22:713–732.

25. Finkelstein RA, Alam HB. Induced hypothermia for trauma: current research and practice. *J Intensive Care Med*. 2010;25:205–226.

26. Wang Q, Li AL, Zhi DS, et al. Effect of mild hypothermia on glucose metabolism and glycerol of brain tissue in patients with severe traumatic brain injury. *Chin J Traumatol*. 2007;10:246–249.

27. Mori M, Maeda M, Miyazaki M, et al. Effects of mild and moderate hypothermia on cerebral metabolism and glutamate in an experimental head injury. *Acta Neurochir Suppl.* 1998;71:222–224.
28. Marion DW, Penrod LE, Kelsey SF, et al. Treatment of traumatic brain injury with moderate hypothermia. *N Engl J Med.* 1997;336:540–546.
29. Metz C, Holzschuh M, Bein T, et al. Moderate hypothermia in patients with severe head injury: cerebral and extracerebral effects. *J Neurosurg.* 1996;85:53–141.
30. Bernard SA, Gray TW, Buist MD, et al. Treatment of comatose survivors of out-of-hospital cardiac arrest with induced hypothermia. *N Engl J Med.* 2002;346:557–563.
31. Hypothermia After Cardiac Arrest Study Group. Mild therapeutic hypothermia to improve the neurologic outcome after cardiac arrest. *N Engl J Med.* 2002;346:549–556.
32. Eicher DJ, Wagner CI, Katikaneni LP, et al. Moderate hypothermia in neonatal encephalopathy: efficacy outcomes. *Pediatr Neurol.* 2005;32:11–17.
33. Gluckman PD, Wyatt JS, Azzopardi D, et al. Selective head cooling with mild systemic hypothermia after neonatal encephalopathy: multicenter randomized trial. *Lancet.* 2005;365: 663–670.
34. Shankaran S, Laptook AR, Ehrenkranz RA, et al. Whole-body hypothermia for neonates with hypoxic-ischemic encephalopathy. *N Engl J Med.* 2005;353:1574–1584.
35. Clasen RA, Pandolfi S, Russell J, et al. Hypothermia and hypotension in experimental cerebral edema. *Arch Neurol.* 1968;19:472–486.
36. Laskowki EJ, Klatzo I, Baldwin M. Experimental study of the effects of hypothermia on local brain injury. *Neurology.* 1960;10:499–505.
37. Rosomoff HL, Gilbert R. Brain volume and cerebrospinal fluid pressure during hypothermia. *Ann J Physiol.* 1955;183:19–22.
38. Rosomoff HL, Shulman K, Raynor R, et al. Experimental brain injury and delayed hypothermia. *Surg Gynecol Observ.* 1960;110:27–32.
39. Ghajar J. Traumatic brain injury. *Lancet.* 2000;356:923–929.
40. Sandestig A, Romner B, Grande P. Therapeutic hypothermia in children and adults with severe traumatic brain injury. *Ther Hypothermia Temp Manag.* 2014;4(1):10–20.
41. Clifton GL, Miller ER, Choi SC, et al. Lack of effect of induction of hypothermia after acute brain injury. *N Engl J Med.* 2001;344:556–563.
42. Andrews PJD, Sinclair LH, Harris B, et al. Study of therapeutic hypothermia (32 to 35°C) for intracranial pressure reduction after traumatic brain injury (the Eurotherm 3235 Trial): outcome of the pilot phase of the trial. *Trials.* 2013;14:277–283.
43. Gasser S, Khan N, Yonekawa Y, et al. Long-term hypothermia in patients with severe brain edema and intensive care complications. *J Neurosurg Anesthesiol.* 2003;15:240–248.
44. Jalan R, Damink SW, Duetz NE, et al. Moderate hypothermia for uncontrolled intracranial hypertension in acute liver failure. *Lancet.* 1999;354:1164–1168.
45. Jalan R, Damink SW, Deutz NE, et al. Moderate hypothermia in patients with acute liver failure and uncontrolled intracranial hypertension. *Gastroenterology.* 2004;127:1338–1346.
46. Schwab S, Georgiadis D, Berrouschot J, et al. Feasibility and safety of moderate hypothermia after massive hemispheric infarction. *Stroke.* 2001;32:2033–2035.
47. Badjatia N. Fever control in the neuro ICU: why, who and when? *Crit Care Med.* 2009;15:79–82.
48. Prasad K, Krishnan PR. Fever is associated with doubling of odds of short-term mortality in ischemic stroke: an updated meta-analysis. *Acta Neurol Scand.* 2010;122:404–408.
49. Fernandez A, Schmidt DM, Claassen J, et al. Fever after subarachnoid hemorrhage. *Neurology.* 2007;68:1013–1019.

50. Springer MV, Schmidt JM, Wartenberg KE, et al. Predictors of global cognitive impairment 1 year after subarachnoid hemorrhage. *Neurosurgery*. 2009;65:1043–1051.

51. McIlvoy L. Fever management in patients with brain injury. *AACN Adv Crit Care*. 2012;23(2):204–211.

52. Reith J, Jorgensen HS, Pedersen PM, et al. Body temperature in acute stroke: relations to stroke severity, infarct size, mortality, and outcome. *Lancet*. 1996;347:422–425.

53. Oliveira-Filho J, Ezzeddine MA, Segal AZ, et al. Fever in subarachnoid hemorrhage: relationship to vasospasm and outcome. *Neurology*. 2001;56:1299–1304.

54. Schwarz S, Hafner K, Aschoff A, et al. Incidence and prognostic significance of fever following intracerebral hemorrhage. *Neurology*. 2000;54:354–361.

55. Chmayssani M, Stein NR, McArthur DL, et al. Therapeutic intravascular normothermia reduces the burden of metabolic crisis. *Neurocrit Care*. 2015;22:265–272.

56. Puccio AM, Fischer MR, Jankowitz BT, et al. Induced normothermia attenuates intracranial hypertension and reduces fever burden after severe traumatic brain injury. *Neurocrit Care*. 2009;11:82–87.

57. Tomte O, Draegni T, Mangschau A, et al. A comparison of intravascular and surface cooling techniques in comatose cardiac arrest survivors. *Crit Care Med*. 2011;39(3): 443–449.

58. Miller CM, Hill M. *Targeted Temperature Management in Acute Neurologic Injury*. AKH Inc .com; no date. AKHcme.com/ttm. Accessed May 14, 2015]

59. Clifton GL, Allen SJ, Berry J, et al. Systemic hypothermia in treatment of brain injury. *J Neurotrauma*. 1992;9(suppl 2):S487–495.

60. Tokutomi T, Morimoto K, Miyagi T, et al. Optimal temperature for the management of traumatic brain injury: effect of hypothermia on intracranial pressure, systemic and intracranial hemodynamics, and metabolism. *Neurosurgery*. 2003;52:102–111.

61. McIntyre LA, Fergusson DA, Hebert PC, et al. Prolonged therapeutic hypothermia after traumatic brain injury in adults: a systematic review. *JAMA*. 2003;289(22):2992–2999.

62. Aslam AF, Aslam AK, Vasavada BC, et al. Hypothermia: evaluation, electrocardiographic manifestations, and management. *Am J Med*. 2006;119:297–301.

63. Choi HA, Ko SB, Presciutti M, et al. Prevention of shivering during therapeutic temperature modulation: the Columbia anti-shivering protocol. *Neurocrit Care*. 2011;14: 389–394.

64. Hildebrand F, Giannoudis PV, van Griensven M, et al. Pathophysiologic changes and effects of hypothermia on outcome in elective surgery and trauma patients. *Am J Surg*. 2004;187:363–371.

65. Clifton GL, Miller ER, Choi SC, et al. Lack of effect of induction of hypothermia after acute brain injury. *N Engl J Med*. 2001;344(8):556–563.

66. Polderman KH. Mechanism of action, physiological effects, and complications of hypothermia. *Crit Care Med*. 2009;37(7):S186–202.

67. Tortorici MA, Kochanek PM, Poloyac SM. Effects of hypothermia on drug disposition, metabolism, and response: a focus of hypothermia-mediated alterations on the cytochrome P450 enzyme system. *Crit Care Med*. 2007;35:2196–2204.

68. Kakashima K, Todd MM, Warner DS. The relation between cerebral metabolic rate and ischemic depolarization. *Anesthesiology*. 1995;82:1199–1208.

69. Chesnut RM, Rondina C, Videtta W, et al. A trial of intracranial pressure monitoring in traumatic brain injury. *N Engl J Med*. 2012;26(26):2471–2481.

70. Nordstrom CH. Volume-targeted therapy of increased intracranial pressure. *Acta Neurochir Suppl*. 2003;86:355–360.

71. Gopinath SP, Robertson CS, Contant CF, et al. Jugular venous desaturation and outcome after head injury. *J Neurol Neurosurg Psychiatry*. 1994;57:717–723.

72. LeRoux PD, Newell DW, Lam AM, et al. Cerebral arteriovenous oxygen difference: a predictor of cerebral infarction and outcome in patients with severe head injury. *J Neurosurg*. 1997;87:1–8.

73. Van Santbrink H, Brink WA, Steyerberg EW, et al. Brain tissue oxygen response in severe traumatic brain injury. *Acta Neurochir* (Vienna). 2003;145:429–438.

7

The Surgical Management of Intracranial Hypertension and Cerebral Herniation Syndromes

Shelly D. Timmons

INTRODUCTION

Surgical approaches to the herniation syndromes can be as varied and distinct as the pathophysiology prompting intervention. The key to avoiding complications and enhancing outcome is to tailor the surgical approach to the problem at hand while still adhering to basic surgical principles and standards of technique. One of the foundations of managing structural traumatic brain injury (TBI) is the appropriate evacuation of mass lesions to remove mass effect and relieve herniation. Additionally, decompressive surgical techniques may allow for cerebral edema egress through the calvarial defect rather than inward, which can result in a herniation syndrome. Combination approaches are the most common in the setting of trauma. Decompressive surgery may also be employed in other scenarios such as ischemic stroke and spontaneous intracerebral hemorrhage.

SURGICAL APPROACHES TO INTRACRANIAL HYPERTENSION AND CEREBRAL HERNIATION

Traumatic Lesions

A surgeon must first consider whether the approach is to treat a focal injury, a global injury, or a combination thereof. Approaches to focal injuries must be anatomically centered over the lesion and directed toward the expedient removal of mass effect with a minimal disruption of surrounding tissues. Approaches to global injuries are by definition larger surgical approaches and must be carefully planned from the beginning. There is no worse intraoperative event than the unexpected complication of brain herniation out of the craniotomy defect, and a lack of preparedness for such an event can be disastrous. During surgery for intracranial hemorrhages and cerebral edema, a failure to plan appropriately can lead to intraoperative catastrophe in the form of brain tissue loss, affecting function, or death.

Leading causes of in-hospital mortality following TBI in the past have included brain edema, elevated intracranial pressure (ICP), and decreased cerebral perfusion pressure. With more aggressive approaches in recent decades, mortality has significantly declined, but these processes can worsen secondary cerebral injury, leading to long-term morbidity. Primary goals for the management of TBI therefore remain to control brain edema and to maintain adequate cerebral perfusion and oxygenation to the cerebral parenchyma. The presence of intracranial mass lesions of all kinds, both traumatic and nontraumatic, can affect edema formation, cause various herniation syndromes depending upon location, and prohibit adequate focal or global cerebral blood flow (CBF) and oxygenation.

Intracranial hemorrhages are commonly associated with severe TBI, ie, those presenting with a Glasgow Coma Scale (GCS) score of 3 to 8. Traumatic hemorrhagic mass lesions include epidural hematoma (EDH) (Figure 7.1), subdural hematoma (SDH) (Figure 7.2), and contusion and intraparenchymal hematoma (IPH).

A contusion may consist of small amounts of blood interspersed with brain tissue or may coalesce into a bona fide hematoma. Traumatic subarachnoid hemorrhage (tSAH), while quite common, is not a surgical problem, and

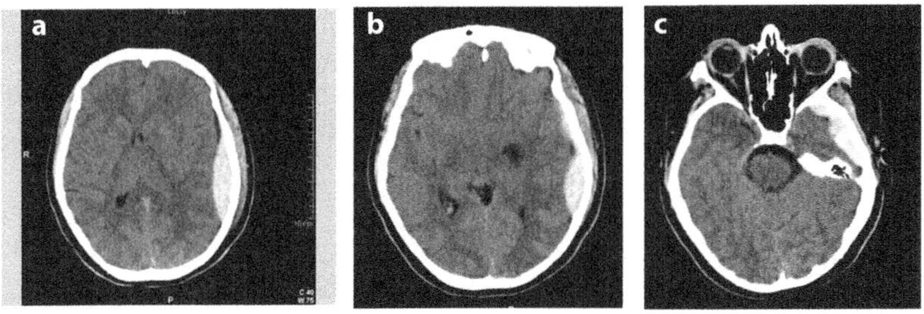

FIGURE 7.1 Epidural hematoma. Note the entrapment of the ipsilateral temporal horn from mass effect and the midline shift.

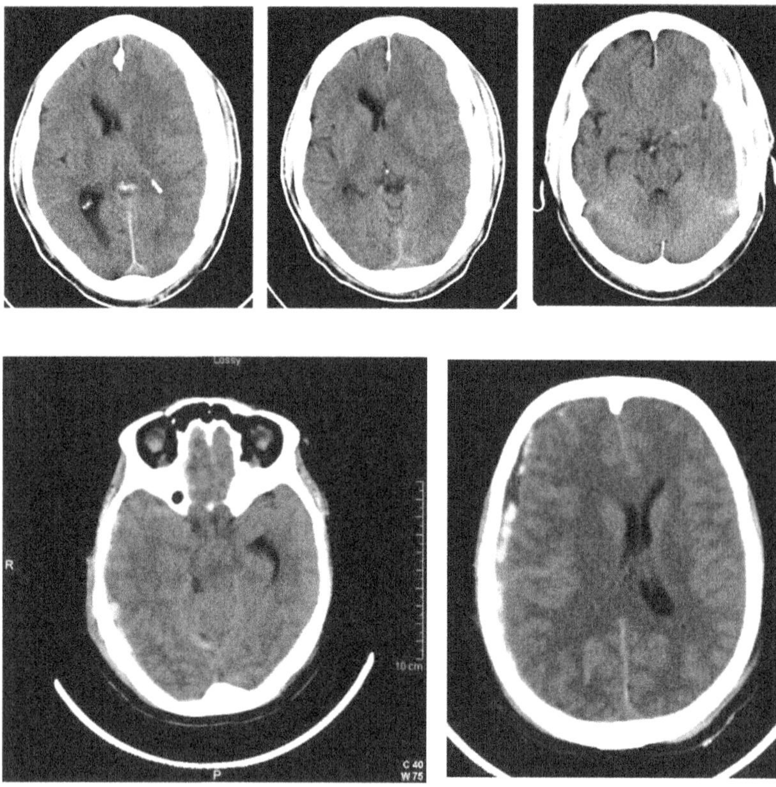

FIGURE 7.2 Subdural hematoma (SDH). Note the differences in the two scans, top row, with midline shift proportional to the SDH and bottom row, midline shift out of proportion to the thickness of the subdural hematoma, signifying hemispheric edema. Note the effaced cisterns and contralateral trapped temporal horn in bottom row that is greater than in top row. These are radiographic signs of cerebral herniation.

neither is the more unusual intraventricular hemorrhage (IVH) unless cerebrospinal fluid (CSF) diversion is required. Evidence-based guidelines for surgery on TBIs were published in 2006 (1). Although many areas of inquiry found insufficient evidence, several major conclusions were drawn from these guidelines and are summarized in Table 7.1.

Decompressive Craniotomy or Craniectomy

Decompressive craniotomy or craniectomy (DC) has long been established as an effective means of decreasing ICP. With the use of DC earlier in the treatment course and advances in neurocritical care management, DC has resulted

TABLE 7.1 Relative indications for the surgical evacuation of traumatic mass lesions

Lesion Type	Clinical Findings	Size/Location of Lesion	Midline Shift	Timing	Type of Surgery
Epidural Hematoma	• Anisocoria referable to lesion AND coma (GCS ≤8) • Focal deficit referable to lesion	• 30 mL regardless of GCS • ≥15 mm thick • Frontal and temporal fossa lower threshold	• ≥5 mm	• ASAP	• Craniotomy
Subdural Hematoma	• GCS ≤8 • GCS decreases by ≥2 points between injury and arrival • Anisocoria • Fixed and dilated pupils • ICP >20 mmHg	• ≥10 mm thick regardless of GCS • ≤10 mm thickness if GCS decreases by ≥2 points between injury and arrival • Anisocoria • Fixed and dilated pupils • ICP >20mmHG	• ≥5 mm Regardless of GCS • ≤5 mm if GCS decreases by ≥2 points between injury and arrival • Anisocoria • Fixed and dilated pupils • ICP >20mmHG	• ASAP	• Craniotomy without bone flap removal • Craniotomy with bone flap removal (midline shift out of proportion to thickness of SDH or other signs of cerebral edema
Intraparen-chymal Hematoma	• Signs of progressive neurological deterioration referable to lesion • Medically refractory elevated ICP	• Mass effect from lesion on CT • GCS 6–8 with frontal or temporal lesion >50 mL • GCS 6–8 with frontal or temporal lesion >20 mL • AND one of the following: • MLS ≥ 5 mm OR • Cisternal effacement	• See size reference	• ASAP	• Craniotomy • Evacuation of hematoma
Multiple Lesions	• Medically refractory ICP • Medically refractory ICP and diffuse parenchymal injury with clinical or radiographic evidence of impending transtentorial herniation			• ASAP	• Decompressive hemicraniotomy/hemicraniectomy • Decompressive bifrontal craniotomy/craniectomy • Subtemporal craniectomy • Temporal lobectomy
Posterior Fossa Hematoma	• Neurological dysfunction • Neurological deterioration	• Mass Effect • Distortion, dislocation, or obliteration of fourth ventricle • Cisternal effacement • Obstructive hydrocephalus		• ASAP	• Wide Suboccipital craniectomy

Source: Adapted from Bullock MR, Chesnut R, Ghajar J, et al. Guidelines for the surgical management of traumatic brain injury author group. *Neurosurgery*. 2006;58:S2.

Note: GCS, Glasgow Coma Scale; ICP, intracranial pressure; MLS, midline shift; SDH, subdural hematoma.

in improved outcomes for severe TBI, stroke, and patients suffering from other maladies. When deciding to use this technique, neurosurgeons should consider, among other things, the preoperative CT findings; the mechanism of injury; and clinical factors such as ICP, cerebral perfusion pressure, and postresuscitation GCS score (particularly the motor component).

Craniotomy is defined as any operation on the cranium, ie, a cut or opening in the skull, whereas craniectomy is defined as an excision of part of the skull. Decompressive cranial surgery for brain swelling or intracranial hypertension in fact incorporates elements of both. It is not strictly a craniectomy because the largest portion of skull removed is eventually replaced. Done properly, however, bone is in fact resected from the temporal fossa in order to achieve adequate decompression of the temporal lobe(s) and relieve uncal herniation. Decompression may incorporate a frontotemporoparietal (FTP) bone flap, a frontotemporoparietooccipital (FTPO) bone flap—either of which is often referred to as a *hemicraniectomy*—or a bifrontal (BF) or bicoronal (BC) bone flap.

Although ICP monitoring and the nonsurgical management of intracranial hypertension may prevent the deleterious effects of diffuse cerebral edema (with or without focal hemorrhage) in many patients, there remains a subset of patients for whom ICP elevation becomes intractable despite maximal medical therapy. These patients are potential candidates for DC in conjunction with evacuation of a hematoma or for primary DC (ie, surgery done specifically to expand the cranial vault and relieve ICP elevation). Both the degree of midline shift and the finding of absent or compressed cisterns on CT of the brain are inversely related to outcome (2). Therefore, patients with major midline shift (generally defined as ≥ 5 mm) and cisternal compromise must be carefully managed and considered for early surgery.

Choice of Technique

Decompressive cranial surgery techniques are employed for trauma in two scenarios, and these can be separated into three broad categories. The first scenario involves planning for and leaving the bone flap out during emergent surgery for an evacuable mass lesion upon presentation. The second scenario is a DC performed later in the hospital course for the treatment of elevated ICP refractory to medical treatment, either with or without the evacuation of mass lesions.

Many hemicraniectomy procedures are done emergently upon presentation when patients have mass lesions (most commonly SDHs) that must be evacuated as a lifesaving procedure. In such cases, radiographic clues must be taken into account to prepare to widely decompress the hemisphere, with the option or intent to perform duraplasty and leave the bone flap out at the end of the operation (see Figure 7.2).

These clues include midline shift out of proportion to the maximum thickness of the SDH, ipsilateral brain edema and/or large contusion burden, ipsilateral cisternal effacement, bilateral obliteration of cisterns, contralateral trapped temporal horn of the lateral ventricle, uncal herniation, subfalcine herniation, early signs of posterior cerebral artery (PCA) distribution ischemia from herniation, or ipsilateral blunt vascular injury, especially carotid injury. Blunt carotid artery injuries are often diagnosed in the current era on computed tomographic angiography (CTA), and their presentation and diagnosis typically precedes the development of ischemic findings on CT. However, subtle findings of well-demarcated vascular territory edema, the loss of sulcal markings, and/or the loss of gray-white junction may be seen even early after a carotid or vertebral artery occlusion or dissection.

Clinical predictors for major brain edema include: ipsilateral or bilateral dilated or unreactive pupil, ipsilateral (Kernohan's notch phenomenon) or contralateral motor deficit (hemiparesis or posturing), bilateral posturing, or the presence of known hypoxia or hypotension in the field or emergency department. Brain matter extrusion from open depressed skull fractures or penetrating wounds presumes major hemispheric injury as well. Finally, the mechanism of injury must be considered. High-velocity mechanisms are more likely to result in global brain injury (with or without focal lesions) than low-velocity mechanisms.

If any of these radiographic or clinical factors are present, the surgeon must be prepared to perform a large incision, large craniotomy, wide hemispheric decompression, temporal craniectomy, and duraplasty with the bone flap left out and stored in a tissue bank, freezer, or the patient's abdominal wall. In cases of gross contamination and/or fragmentation from a comminuted skull fracture, the surgeon must also be prepared to formalize the cranial opening and discard the bone. The decision must be made as to laterality and whether or not to remove any, select, or all mass lesions based upon the examination and CT findings. Intraoperatively, if the findings are not congruent with major hemispheric edema and the brain is well contained within the cranial vault, relaxed, and of normal consistency after evacuation of the lesion, the bone flap can simply be replaced.

The second important clinical scenario is a DC performed to treat elevated ICP refractory to medical treatment. For patients with mass lesions not initially evacuated due to a failure to meet evacuation criteria and good ICP control via medical means who subsequently deteriorate to an uncontrollable ICP situation, repeat CT scanning is generally selected. A decision must then be made again as to surgical laterality and whether or not to remove any, select, or all mass lesions, again based upon the examination and CT findings.

For patients with mass lesions that were not initially evacuated but then enlarge significantly, the enlarging mass lesion will typically be evacuated with or without other lesions depending upon their location, accessibility, and contribution to the overall herniation syndrome.

For patients with no discernible mass lesions (with or without tSAH, IVH, or "salt and pepper" or punctate contusions) and/or those with global hypoxic or shear injury patterns, primary decompression may be selected. If any laterality to the radiographic findings signifies that one hemisphere is more damaged or swollen than the other, the author will typically opt for a hemicranial approach on the more damaged side. If there are no lateralized findings—a notable minority of patients—then a BF approach would be selected with ligation of the anterior superior sagittal sinus, duraplasty, and bilateral temporal craniectomies.

Patient Selection

Older literature from the pre-CT era cites bilaterally fixed and dilated pupils, a GCS score of 3 (without sedating drugs or paralytics on board), brainstem injury, and central herniation as harbingers of a poor outcome after DC (3,4). Indeed, with CT in common usage today, these findings remain negative prognostic indicators. The postresuscitation GCS score, particularly the motor component, remains one of the most important factors to consider in patient selection (5,6). Younger patients generally have better outcomes after a DC (7,8). The decision to proceed with a DC must therefore take these findings into account, as well as the patient's overall medical status, comorbidities, hemodynamic state, and degree of polytrauma.

Patient wishes and personal definitions of a meaningful life and recovery must always be considered when providing therapeutic options to families. However, predictions of outcome in the early phases after injury are notoriously poor (9), and accurate prognostication can be difficult. Caution must be taken against the self-fulfilling prophecy of assuming futility in the early phases after TBI, as failing to treat prolonged intracranial hypertension is nearly universally fatal—and if not fatal, highly contributory to a poor outcome.

Rationale and Evidence Basis

The timing of surgery is equally important. Mortality increases when ICP is not controlled (10–12). Marmarou et al demonstrated the correlation of total time of ICP elevation and outcome with the Traumatic Coma Data Bank of the 1980s (13). In the very early days of CT, it was recognized that an abnormal CT scan (the presence of high- or low-density lesions) at admission is predictive of high ICP, and of those with normal scans upon admission, the presence of two or more of the following features are predictive of high ICP: an age over 40, an episode of hypotension (systolic blood pressure [SBP] < 90 mmHg), or motor posturing (14). The guidelines for ICP monitoring in TBI are largely based upon this landmark study. Well over half (69%) of patients who died from severe TBI in one large study in the 1990s died from "increased intracranial volume" causing high ICP (15). The incidence of ICP elevation requiring therapy in a severe TBI cohort is estimated at 65% (16).

Knowing that patients with mass lesions after TBI are at high risk for intracranial hypertension and that its presence, especially if prolonged, is associated with increased mortality, consideration must be given to early surgery to remove mass lesions and relieve high ICP. Numerous studies conducted since these seminal articles were published have shown that outcomes improve after early surgery. Therefore, patients should not be allowed to languish for hours or days with high ICP prior to surgery. A DC should be considered once medical therapy fails to control ICP.

The definition of the failure of medical therapy may vary from patient to patient depending upon other physiological parameters. Patients with modest ICP elevations but adequate cerebral perfusion pressure, CBF, lactate to pyruvate ratios, and/or brain tissue oxygenation ($PbtO_2$) may not require surgery. Patients may tolerate this situation for a longer amount of time than sustained very high ICP elevations. Conversely, patients with impairments in other neuromonitoring parameters, such as CPP, CBF, $PbtO_2$, or lactate to pyruvate ratios, and only modest elevations in ICP may benefit from surgery.

Over the past 30 years, more than 20 centers have published retrospective or nonrandomized prospective case studies (class II and III evidence) on outcomes in patients undergoing DC for multiple causes, with a mean mortality rate of 20% to 30%, as opposed to 70% to 80% in patients treated conservatively (31). However, wide variability exists in reported outcomes in the literature, which may be ascribed to a lack of standardization of technique, a lack of standardization of medical management, a lack of standardized outcomes procedures, heterogeneity in patient groups, a lack of a control group, and intercenter variability from other causes. More recent studies have used DC as an earlier treatment option for controlling ICP, and numerous authors have demonstrated improved outcomes (both for mortality and functional outcome) with DC for severe TBI (6,8,17–22).

Two recent multicenter, prospective randomized controlled trials of DC in patients with severe diffuse TBI are of note: the Australian Decompressive Craniectomy in Diffuse Traumatic Brain Injury trial (DECRA) (23) and the international Randomised Evaluation of Surgery With Craniectomy for

Uncontrollable Elevation of ICP (RESCUEicp) trial (24). These trials had different designs. The DECRA trial took place over approximately 7.5 years and included 155 adult patients with severe diffuse TBI (ie, without mass lesions). Patients were randomized to bifrontotemporoparietal DC without ligation of the superior sagittal sinus or standard medical care, and crossover was allowed. The Extended Glasgow Outcome Score (GOS-E) 6 months after injury was used to measure primary outcome. The RESCUEicp trial examined pediatric and adult patients, also over a number of years, with and without evacuable mass lesions and contusions, and utilized hemicraniectomy techniques. This study utilized a higher threshold both in ICP measurements and the duration of ICP elevation prior to randomization to surgery. Outcome assessments included 6-, 12-, and 24-month GOS-E and the Short Form 36 Health Survey (SF-36) quality of life measure. The RESCUEicp study has closed enrollment, and the results are being analyzed.

Ischemic Stroke

Patients with ischemic infarction may also benefit from a DC. Predictors of malignant cerebral edema after a stroke include a National Institutes of Health Stroke Score (NIHSS) greater than 20, thrombus at the carotid terminus, nausea and/or vomiting, an elevated white blood cell count, early involvement of greater than 50% of the middle cerebral artery (MCA) territory on CT scan, additional involvement of the anterior cerebral artery (ACA) and/or the PCA territories, anterior choroidal artery (AChA) involvement, and/or uncal herniation (25). Several clinical trials have been conducted in order to help identify those patients who would benefit most from surgical decompression, including the Decompressive Surgery for the Treatment of Malignant Infarction of the Middle Cerebral Artery (DESTINY) trial, the Decompressive Craniectomy in Malignant Middle Cerebral Artery Infarction (DECIMAL) trial, the Hemicraniectomy After Middle Cerebral Artery Infarction With Life-Threatening Edema trial (HAMLET), and DESTINY II (26–29). An age less than 60 years is a relative indication for surgery, as is a severe MCA distribution infarction with an NIHSS greater than 15. However, a subsequent study (DESTINY II) eliminated age as a criterion because older patients fared well, so recommendations currently do not include an upper age "limit." Older patients with a greater degree of atrophy can accommodate larger infarct volumes without experiencing herniation from cerebral edema, whereas malignant edema will result in brainstem compression in younger patients. Young patients with very large infarct volumes are therefore at high risk of rapid deterioration and death within the first 48 hours, and decompressive surgery can save these patients' lives but does not reduce stroke-associated deficits. As per prior discussion, family and patient wishes must be taken into account when deciding on a surgery that will increase survival without improving deficits in patients of advanced age.

Neurological decline and drowsiness can be defined as an NIHSS 1A level of consciousness change greater than or equal to 1 point or a GCS eye-opening and motor response subtotal less than or equal to 9. If the infarct volume is greater than 50% of the MCA territory or the total infarct volume is greater than 145 cm^3, surgery may also be beneficial. Finally, the timing of surgery is important for its success, and in general, patients who are referred within 24 hours of ischemic stroke onset and/or who undergo decompressive surgery within 48 hours of onset fare better. A recent meta-analysis of the DESTINY, DECIMAL, and HAMLET trials demonstrated similar outcomes after DC in dominant and nondominant hemisphere strokes (30).

COMMON ADVERSE EFFECTS AND PREVENTION TECHNIQUES

No surgical approach is without the potential for complications and adverse events. Common problems after a DC can be broadly broken down into the following categories: (a) CSF dynamics, (b) cerebral complications, (c) wound problems, and (d) other technique-related issues.

Cerebrospinal Fluid Dynamics

CSF dynamic issues include the formation of hygromas (benign CSF collection) and other alterations in CSF flow or absorption, including hydrocephalus (low and high pressure). Hydrocephalus can occur before and after staged secondary bone flap replacement after a DC. In essence, these problems may occur with or without any surgical procedure after trauma, but removing the cranial flap may alter the course, and several nuances in management must be considered.

First, it must be understood that at least some degree of hygroma formation is nearly universal after a DC, occurring most frequently ipsilateral to the DC (6). Hygroma formation is arguably defined as a complication since there is no clinical consequence in most instances. Typically, hygromas resolve spontaneously without intervention, but some may require percutaneous drainage, serial lumbar puncture, a course of lumbar drainage, or extracranial shunting (31). Frequently, hygroma(s) will resolve after replacing the bone flap. In the author's experience, suturing the duraplasty graft in place and restoring the dural integrity, especially if achieving a watertight or near-watertight closure, reduces the formation of peripheral hygromas (both incidence and size).

Hydrocephalus may occur preoperatively or postoperatively and must be distinguished from *hydrocephalus ex vacuo*, or ventricular dilation due to encephalomalacia and cerebral volume loss. Hydrocephalus may be low pressure or high pressure and is typically—though not exclusively—communicating, meaning that an obstruction does not isolate the ventricular chambers from one another. Treatment options for true hydrocephalus include serial lumbar punctures to restore CSF flow in the face of high protein and high cellular contents from the breakdown of blood products, a trial of lumbar drainage for the same purpose, or temporary external ventricular CSF drainage. Failing all such efforts to restore CSF circulation, permanent extracranial shunting may be necessary. If this is required, the type of valve (low, medium, or high pressure), the use of antisiphon devices, or the use of a programmable valve, as well as the distal drainage site (peritoneum, pleural space, or cardiac atrium) must be carefully considered. This consideration should be based upon an understanding of the CSF dynamics assessments done previously, the current CSF laboratory values (protein and cellularity), and the patient's expected functional level (primarily upright or supine).

The most opportune time for shunting may vary from patient to patient. Patients who repeatedly have ventricular dilation resulting in brain herniation through the cranial defect may require shunting prior to or simultaneous to replacing the bone flap. The risk for infection later in the course must be assessed for both the shunt and the bone flap. For mild ventricular dilation, replacing the bone flap and carefully observing the ventricular size with serial CT scanning may help avoid a postoperative shunt. Conversely, if a neurological change and/or excessive dilation of ventricles over and above that expected from encephalomalacia occur, a shunt may be needed after bone flap replacement. The surgeon must also take into account the timing from injury, the degree of persistent cerebral hemorrhage, the degree of persistent cerebral edema, and the potential for ongoing injury to the cerebral tissue if the hemisphere is allowed to expand and herniate out of the cranial defect (edge contusion/ischemia/edema). Chronic low-grade hydrocephalus may manifest in wound breakdown and a CSF leak or bone flap resorption from ICP.

In summary, the most frequently encountered complications of DC reported in the literature include hydrocephalus (14%–29%) and hygroma formation (24%–50%) (6,31,32). Deciding when and how to treat posttraumatic hydrocephalus in the setting of DC is sometimes quite complex. The surgeon must take a thoughtful approach to these problems and consider the evolution of the brain injury and its radiographic appearance over time, the patient's ICP history and dynamic responses to intervention, CSF laboratory values, and plans for bone flap replacement, including timing. A CT of the head should be obtained just prior to the staged secondary bone flap replacement to assess the ventricular system, to note the presence of hygroma formation (which can possibly be drained at surgery if needed), and to assess the degree of positive or negative midline shift and hemispheric positioning relative to the edges of the bony defect. If the brain and/or the ventricular system are slightly "full," the surgeon may consider placing an intraoperative lumbar drain to aid in relaxation for bone flap replacement.

Cerebral Complications

Problems related to the brain itself include the *syndrome of the trephined*, seizures, progression of contusion and hematoma, and border ischemia and hemorrhages (with or without improper technique).

Grant and Norcross described the syndrome of the trephined in 1939 as a condition characterized by headaches, dizziness, mood changes, or seizures in patients who had undergone a DC (33). Focal neurological deficits may also occur. The progression toward earlier and earlier replacement of the bone flap, in many cases 8 to 12 weeks postoperatively (instead of the 6- to 12-month delays commonplace in past decades), has reduced the incidence of this syndrome. The early low-functioning patient who is discharged to a skilled-nursing facility without early follow-up is at risk. As the brain becomes encephalomalacic, the flap sinks, and not only does a pressure differential occur between the intracranial contents and the atmosphere, but the scalp can also contract, placing direct traction on the brain. The neurological status may improve with surgical correction of this syndrome.

Although the long-term consequences of limited seizure activity on functional outcome are not well defined, seizures can lead to potential negative outcomes from status epilepticus or increased ICP, contributing to herniation syndromes, and should be avoided and treated aggressively in the acute phases of all types of brain injuries. Seizures can occur in both the acute and chronic phases after a DC, with persistent seizure activity in up to 5% of patients undergoing a DC for trauma (31). Evidence-based guidelines should be used for decision making after acute trauma. For severe TBI, the guidelines include a level II recommendation for decreasing the incidence of early posttraumatic seizures. The use of 7 days of prophylactic medication is supported for SDH, EDH, contusion or IPH, a penetrating brain injury, a depressed skull fracture, a GCS score less than 10, or an immediate or early posttraumatic seizure (within

24 hours of injury) (34). Its use in isolated traumatic SAH and intraventricular hemorrhage is not supported. The choice of agent should be based upon the literature as well as patient factors. Studies supporting the guidelines include the use of phenytoin and valproic acid. The side-effect profile of phenytoin (Dilantin) in severely brain-injured patients is low. Adverse effects that can occur even at therapeutic doses, such as drowsiness and ataxia, are not clinically relevant to the patient in a coma. "Dilantin rash" and the rarely occurring Stevens-Johnson syndrome are unusual with such short courses of therapy. Finally, the cost of the agent should be considered in high-volume trauma settings. Most of the novel anticonvulsants are not only unproven for this treatment scenario but also much more costly.

Seizures can occur in up to 20% of aneurysmal SAH patients, usually within the first 24 hours. The incidence is higher in those with associated intracerebral hemorrhage, MCA aneurysms, or hypertension (35). Although the guidelines currently recommend anticonvulsants, they stand moot on the choice of agent (27). Routine long-term use is not recommended, and a recent study suggests that just 72 hours of therapy is adequate (36). For ischemic infarction, their utility is less clear. Other entities that may rarely require a DC, such as arteriovenous malformation hemorrhage or infection, would be treated on a case-by-case basis depending on whether or not the presentation included seizure.

Since seizure prophylaxis after TBI or aneurysmal SAH is not routine after 7 days from injury based on guidelines, most patients are not on anticonvulsants at the time they undergo their bone flap replacement procedure (unless they experience late posttraumatic or posthemorrhage seizures). In the author's extensive experience, the second phase of high risk for seizures is in the hours and days after the staged secondary bone flap replacement surgery. For this reason, the routine use of an intraoperative loading dose (typically with phenytoin) followed by 1 week of seizure prophylaxis has achieved good success in reducing recovery room and early postoperative seizures. If patients are on an anticonvulsant for late seizures, a second agent will be temporarily added in the same fashion.

Technical approaches during the second surgery to help prevent postoperative seizures include avoiding heat transmission from Bovie and bipolar cautery to the underlying brain tissue and avoiding traction on underlying damaged brain tissue, especially the temporal lobe, during dissection of the temporalis muscle off the underlying dura. The author has described a technique to place a subtemporalis barrier with a nonincorporated graft material (in addition to and overlying a sutured duraplasty patch graft that will incorporate with native dura). This subtemporalis barrier facilitates later dissection of the temporalis muscle off the underlying dura, which not only speeds the dissection but requires less tissue manipulation of the typically encephalomalacic and formerly compromised temporal lobe.

Finally, the choice of duraplasty technique at the initial surgery can have an impact on the long-term integrity of cerebral tissue. Although many surgeons choose to employ nonsutured onlay graft techniques, care must be taken when choosing the material and placement technique. When no suture technique is used, the graft can shift as the brain swells and then subsides. This can directly expose the brain to the galeal layer and cause already vulnerable cerebral tissue to adhere to the galea, leading to additional damage during the postoperative period as the scalp expands and contracts, as well as during the subsequent dissection for bone flap replacement. The author's preferred technique is therefore to suture the dura in place, and if closure needs to be expedited, to at least provide tacking sutures in the perimeter of the graft material to prevent migration with overlap of the graft over the edge of the native dura. Both measures will limit the degree of exposed brain.

Cerebral complications also include secondary injury from vascular dynamics. Once the swollen hemisphere decompresses, a reduction in ICP facilitates blood flow. Cerebral vasodilation and hyperemia may then lead to perfusion breakthrough hemorrhage. Conversely, areas at the margins of the bony decompression are particularly vulnerable to venous compression. Both of these phenomena may lead to increased cerebral edema. Avoiding the former is difficult and relies upon neurocritical care management strategies, careful attention to blood pressure, and the use of neuromonitoring technologies. Proper surgical planning helps to avoid the latter. Care must be taken when constructing the opening in the cranial vault to make the opening high where the skull becomes flat (while avoiding the superior sagittal sinus). This way, when the hemisphere swells outward, it swells laterally, and the downward-curving cranial vault does not compress the cerebral draining veins at the upper edge of the cerebral hemisphere. Some have advocated the creation of tunnels or the placement of pledgets around prominent draining veins, but the author has found the technique so described to be sufficient. Similarly, the opening must be carried completely to the floor of the middle fossa to avoid strangulating the brain and cerebral vessels over any remaining wall of squamous temporal bone. Figure 7.3 demonstrates the degree of decompression needed to avoid these pitfalls.

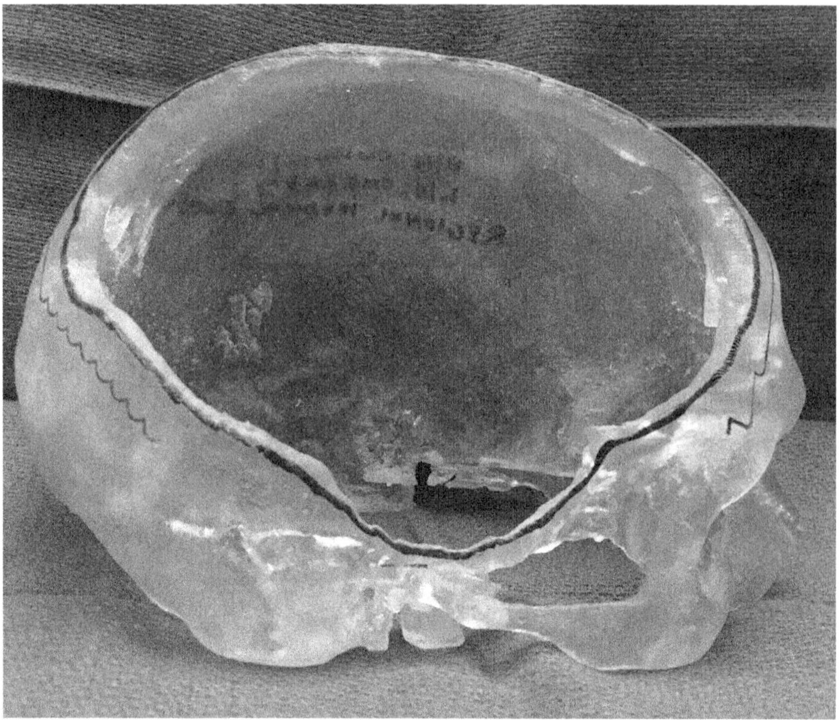

FIGURE 7.3 A model used for construction of a patient-specific cranial implant demonstrating the large size necessary for a decompressive hemicraniectomy and the extent of resection needed to the floor of the temporal fossa.

Wound Complications

Wound complications can occur with even the most meticulous technique. However, it is important to master the technical aspects of this surgery, especially because the initial incision, musculocutaneous bone flap dissection, and craniotomy are performed in emergency circumstances and must be executed quickly while taking later needs into account. Therefore, it pays to think through tissue handling in advance.

Inspecting the head in its entirety is a major element of preparation at initial surgery. Because in the setting of trauma the presence of hair may obscure soft tissue injuries, the author recommends clipping the entire hemicranium, at a minimum. First, the entire scalp must be palpated for lacerations, which should be quickly repaired preoperatively if there is significant bleeding so that occult blood loss under the drapes does not contribute to poor outcome.

Brisk scalp bleeding from traumatic lacerations, especially in the areas of the occipital artery and its branches and the superficial temporal artery (STA) and its branches, can actually lead to the demise of the patient through massive blood loss, hypotension, and cardiovascular collapse, so these must be addressed expeditiously. Even in patients undergoing a DC for other indications, such as stroke, the scalp should be inspected, as catastrophic events leading to cerebral edema can lead to falls and secondary head trauma.

Second, the choice of scalp incision must take into account that the incision will definitely be reopened at least once in the future for survivors, and potentially multiple times. Therefore, attention must be paid to the handling of lacerations, abrasions, hematomas, and blood supply during the preparation. The incision should incorporate deep lacerations and avoid crossing significant lacerations, abrasions, or hematomas if at all possible. The blood supply must be maintained from a vascular pedicle to the flap. Options for incisions include a very large FTPO or FTP standard "question mark" or "reverse question mark" incision. This incision is the author's preference for adequately accessing the temporal fossa floor and the entire hemicranium without undue traction on the scalp from retraction (which can lead to tissue ischemia and later wound breakdown). Other options include a large curvilinear incision from the retroauricular or mastoid area extending to the frontal area. This limits access to the temporal fossa floor, however, and requires extensive temporalis muscle retraction and dissection, which can lead to ischemia and atrophy. On the other hand, the temporalis muscle does not require vertical incisional division because it is primarily subperiosteally dissected off the calvarium. Another option is a "T" incision incorporating a vertical limb anterior to the ear over the temporalis and a large parasagittal incision. This incision provides excellent access to the hemicranium and the hemisphere and the temporal fossa floor but risks poor healing at the junction of the two incisions, especially with repeated openings.

Decubitus ulcers may occur with incisions placed too posteriorly where the patient's head rests on the bed, even with frequent turning and excellent nursing care, so the placement of the incision must be marked to avoid this. The scalp incision should be wider than the craniotomy opening to avoid positioning the bone edge immediately under the incision, which can promote dehiscence as swelling subsides. Likewise, during the secondary bone flap replacement, screws and plates should be placed so that they do not lie directly underneath the incision. Finally, the incision should not be placed too close to the pinna of the ear, as scarring here will often interfere with wearing glasses, can be painful, or may contribute to a poor cosmetic result. A significant cuff of scalp may be left over the pinna, as this is easily retracted to avoid interference with the bone flap creation.

Handling of the temporalis muscle should preserve the STA if possible. Resecting the muscle should be avoided. The muscle fascia is typically left open after duraplasty so as not to allow the muscle to constrict the swelling temporal lobe. Although the temporalis can be left in its dependent position upon bone flap replacement, the muscle is ideally dissected off the dura and placed back on the outside of the bone flap (or artificial implant if used) to not only enhance cosmesis but also to avoid pain with chewing and to prevent a "sagging" protrusion of the muscle that can interfere with wearing glasses.

Suboptimal surgical technique can contribute to wound infection, incisional dehiscence, scalp devitalization, and pinholing. Care to respect the layers of the scalp during opening and to adequately close the galea and skin layers during closure will help avoid these issues. Accessible full-thickness scalp lacerations should be repaired from the inside (galea) and the outside (skin) to facilitate healing. As the initial procedure must often be performed precipitously, the surgeon must be facile at obtaining a good technical opening and closure in an expeditious fashion.

Particularly prone to wound dehiscence are patients with thin scalps (eg, women, the elderly, and patients with irradiated crania), patients with contracted scalps from chronically sunken flaps, the malnourished, and smokers. The patient's nutritional status must be a top priority immediately upon presentation, as patients in coma have greatly increased nutritional requirements. Coma patients should attain full caloric replacement by 7 days postinjury (37), preferably with enteral feedings. In the long term, poor nutritional status will affect wound healing and can contribute to dehiscence, so a full nutritional workup should be considered prior to bone replacement for all patients who lack full function or who are still receiving nutritional supplementation. The potential impact on wound healing from a prior smoking history, prior alcohol consumption, an older age and thinning tissues, physiological stress, diabetes mellitus, steroid administration, and sex hormone imbalance must be assessed (38). For patients with all forms of brain insult, especially TBI and most especially TBI from a frontal impact, an evaluation of the hypothalamic pituitary axis must be considered, as occult derangements in hormone balance may occur and affect wound healing.

Bone flap resorption has been reported in up to 12% of patients after secondary bone flap replacement, with approximately half requiring removal and replacement with a synthetic implant (6). Both hydrocephalus and low-grade infection can lead to bone flap resorption, as previously noted. In the author's experience, the incidence of bone flap resorption also increases in the following scenarios: younger patient age (children, teenagers, and young adults), prolonged freezer storage, irradiation, or a bone flap significantly fragmented by fracture. Reports of resorption during storage in the abdominal wall have also been published.

Resorption typically manifests clinically with a new onset of headache late after replacement, owing most likely to trephination syndrome–style pressure changes. Palpable defects in the cranium or pulsatility in areas of uncovered or thinly covered brain may be noted. The patient may also experience auditory clicking from the threads of free-floating screws and plates. CT scan, especially a thin-cut CT suitable for computer-guided, patient-specific implant (PSI) construction, is the definitive diagnostic tool and the test of choice. Evidence of hydrocephalus or infection that could be contributing factors may show up on this CT. If any question of infection exists, serum laboratory studies may be required.

When resorption is symptomatic or when large areas of cerebrum lie unprotected, the bone flap should be removed and replaced with a PSI. This is often preferred over an intraoperatively manufactured skull reconstruction, owing to the large size of the cranial defect. The use of a PSI is faster intraoperatively and provides better calvarial reconstruction and complete brain coverage with a minimum of effort. These implants are available in a variety of materials, including polyetheretherketone (PEEK), polymethyl methacrylate (PMMA), acrylic, and even solid or meshed titanium.

DC itself does not confer any special susceptibility to infection over the quoted rates of 3% to 5% for standard craniotomy (6,31). Patients presenting postoperatively with new or enlarging subdural or epidural/subgaleal fluid collections should undergo CT of the head with and without contrast to rule out empyema, and appropriate laboratory studies, including a complete blood count with differential, an erythrocyte sedimentation rate, and a measure of C-reactive protein, are useful adjuncts. As noted, special consideration to infection must be given when bone flap resorption is identified, as chronic or low-grade infections can result in this phenomenon.

Prior infection history from the initial hospitalization must always be surveyed, as these critical patients are prone to hospital-acquired infection from a variety of factors. These include immobility from injury and the development of decubitus ulcers; the need for prolonged mechanical ventilation; the need for indwelling urinary catheters to adequately assess and manage fluid balance and disorders common to these patients; and the need for prolonged indwelling vascular access lines, such as central venous catheters and arterial lines, which are also mainstays of assessment and management in the neurocritical care unit. Chest tubes, external fixators, traction devices, and other surgical procedures confer additional infection risk, as do soft tissue injuries from polytrauma. Episodes and durations of ventilator-associated pneumonia; tracheitis; urinary tract infections; bacteremia; septicemia; soft tissue, thoracic, abdomino-pelvic, or limb infections; or infections resulting from other trauma, procedures, or surgeries must be known to the neurosurgical operator, along with the treatment, duration of treatment, and stage of treatment when considering any neurosurgical interventions. Skin surveys should be conducted. These measures will help determine the timing of staged secondary bone flap replacement as well as any other implanted devices, such as ventriculoperitoneal, ventriculopleural, or ventriculoatrial shunts.

For complicated wound dehiscence with secondary infection and for documented cranial infections such as empyema or osteomyelitis, the bone flap must be removed and discarded. A PSI can be used at a future setting (not the surgical setting of removal) once it has been ascertained that the infection has been adequately treated. This often requires prolonged (ie, 6 weeks or more) intravenous antibiotic therapy. Plastic surgery techniques, such as rotational flaps or tissue expansion, are often required for complicated wounds in order to achieve adequate calvarial implant coverage with healthy tissue.

Other Complications

Traction nerve palsy of the frontotemporal branches of the facial nerve can occur with aggressive dissection within the fat pad overlying the temporalis muscle, resulting most commonly in significant frontalis muscle paralysis. The supraorbital nerve can be damaged at the exit in the supraorbital foramen, especially in direct facial trauma or during BC operations, resulting in a loss of sensation to the forehead and the periorbital area.

CONCLUSIONS

The choice of a surgical technique for managing intracranial hypertension and cerebral herniation syndromes is a sophisticated one. DC is a useful surgical adjunct to medically managing TBI and stroke as well as other conditions leading to cerebral edema, such as intracranial aneurysm rupture with hematoma or infarction, spontaneous ICH, and rarer conditions such as intracerebral abscess. The astute neurosurgeon must take into account a plethora of factors, including evidence in the literature for use of DC in certain populations of patients and a wide variety of patient-specific characteristics, in order to optimize survival and ultimately long-term functional outcome after a DC. Attention to surgical planning and the details of technique will avoid most complications, improving the operation's overall risk-to-benefit profile.

Acknowledgment

The author would like to thank the following individuals for contributing reference and other background information to the manuscript: Mayur Jayarao, MD; Clemens M. Schirmer, MD, PhD; and Tarun Bhalla, MD, PhD.

References

1. Bullock MR, Chesnut R, Ghajar J, et al. Guidelines for the surgical management of traumatic brain injury author group. *Neurosurgery*. 2006;58:S2.

2. Eisenberg HM, Gary HE Jr, Aldrich EF, et al. Initial CT findings in 753 patients with severe head injury. A report from the NIH Traumatic Coma Data Bank. *J Neurosurg*. 1990;73:688–698.

3. Gaab MR, Rittierodt M, Lorenz M, et al. Traumatic brain swelling and operative decompression: a prospective investigation. *Acta Neurochir Suppl* (Vienna). 1990;51:326–328.

4. Yamaura A, Uemura K, Makino H. Large decompressive craniectomy in management of severe cerebral contusion. A review of 207 cases. *Neurol Med Chir* (Tokyo). 1979;19:717–728.

5. Woertgen C, Erban P, Rothoerl RD, et al. Quality of life after decompressive craniectomy in patients suffering from supratentorial brain ischemia. *Acta Neurochir* (Vienna). 2004;146:691–695.

6. Aarabi B, Hesdorffer DC, Ahn ES, et al. Outcome following decompressive craniectomy for malignant swelling due to severe head injury. *J Neurosurg*. 2006;104:469–479.

7. Ucar T, Akyuz M, Kazan S, et al. Role of decompressive surgery in the management of severe head injuries: prognostic factors and patient selection. *J Neurotrauma*. 2005;22:1311–1318.

8. Williams RF, Magnotti LJ, Croce MA, et al. Impact of decompressive craniectomy on functional outcome after severe traumatic brain injury. *J Trauma*. 2009;66:1570–1574; (discussion):4–6.

9. Kaufmann MA, Buchmann B, Scheidegger D, et al. Severe head injury: should expected outcome influence resuscitation and first-day decisions? *Resuscitation*. 1992;23:199–206.

10. Saul TG, Ducker TB. Intracranial pressure monitoring in patients with severe head injury. *Am Surg*. 1982;48:477–480.

11. Saul TG, Ducker TB. Effect of intracranial pressure monitoring and aggressive treatment on mortality in severe head injury. *J Neurosurg*. 1982;56:498–503.

12. Eisenberg HM, Frankowski RF, Contant CF, et al. High-dose barbiturate control of elevated intracranial pressure in patients with severe head injury. *J Neurosurg*. 1988;69:15–23.

13. Marmarou A. Increased intracranial pressure in head injury and influence of blood volume. *J Neurotrauma*. 1992;9(suppl 1):S327–332.

14. Narayan RK, Kishore PR, Becker DP, et al. Intracranial pressure: to monitor or not to monitor? A review of our experience with severe head injury. *J Neurosurg*. 1982;56:650–659.

15. Marshall LF, Maas AI, Marshall SB, et al. A multicenter trial on the efficacy of using tirilazad mesylate in cases of head injury. *J Neurosurg*. 1998;89:519–525.

16. Hukkelhoven CW, Steyerberg EW, Farace E, et al. Regional differences in patient characteristics, case management, and outcomes in traumatic brain injury: experience from the tirilazad trials. *J Neurosurg*. 2002;97:549–557.

17. Kontopoulos V, Foroglou N, Patsalas J, et al. Decompressive craniectomy for the management of patients with refractory hypertension: should it be reconsidered? *Acta Neurochir* (Vienna). 2002;144:791–796.

18. Meier U, Zeilinger FS, Henzka O. The use of decompressive craniectomy for the management of severe head injuries. *Acta Neurochir Suppl*. 2000;76:475–478.
19. Polin RS, Shaffrey ME, Bogaev CA, et al. Decompressive bifrontal craniectomy in the treatment of severe refractory posttraumatic cerebral edema. *Neurosurgery*. 1997;41:84–92; (discussion):4.
20. Munch E, Horn P, Schurer L, et al. Management of severe traumatic brain injury by decompressive craniectomy. *Neurosurgery*. 2000;47:315–322;(discussion):22–23.
21. Coplin WM. Intracranial pressure and surgical decompression for traumatic brain injury: biological rationale and protocol for a randomized clinical trial. *Neurol Res*. 2001;23: 277–290.
22. Coplin WM, Cullen NK, Policherla PN, et al. Safety and feasibility of craniectomy with duraplasty as the initial surgical intervention for severe traumatic brain injury. *J Trauma*. 2001;50:1050–1059.
23. Hutchinson P, Timofeev I, Kirkpatrick P. Surgery for brain edema. *Neurosurg Focus*. 2007;22:E14.
24. Hutchinson PJ, Corteen E, Czosnyka M, et al. Decompressive craniectomy in traumatic brain injury: the randomized multicenter RESCUEicp study. *Acta Neurochir Suppl*. 2006;96: 17–20.
25. Staykov D, Gupta R. Hemicraniectomy in malignant middle cerebral artery infarction. *Stroke*. 2011;42:513–516.
26. Juttler E, Bosel J, Amiri H, et al. DESTINY II: Decompressive Surgery for the Treatment of Malignant Infarction of the Middle Cerebral Artery II. *Int J Stroke*. 2011;6: 79–86.
27. Hofmeijer J, Kappelle LJ, Algra A, et al. Surgical decompression for space-occupying cerebral infarction (the Hemicraniectomy After Middle Cerebral Artery Infarction with Life-Threatening Edema Trial [HAMLET]): a multicentre, open, randomised trial. *Lancet Neurol*. 2009;8:326–333.
28. Vahedi K, Vicaut E, Mateo J, et al. Sequential-design, multicenter, randomized, controlled trial of early decompressive craniectomy in malignant middle cerebral artery infarction (DECIMAL trial). *Stroke*. 2007;38:2506–2517.
29. Juttler E, Schwab S, Schmiedek P, et al. Decompressive Surgery for the Treatment of Malignant Infarction of the Middle Cerebral Artery (DESTINY): a randomized, controlled trial. *Stroke*. 2007;38:2518–2525.
30. Vibbert M, Mayer SA. Early decompressive hemicraniectomy following malignant ischemic stroke: the crucial role of timing. *Curr Neurol Neurosci Rep*. 2010;10:1–3.
31. Guerra WK, Gaab MR, Dietz H, et al. Surgical decompression for traumatic brain swelling: indications and results. *J Neurosurg*. 1999;90:187–196.
32. Chibbaro S, Tacconi L. Role of decompressive craniectomy in the management of severe head injury with refractory cerebral edema and intractable intracranial pressure. Our experience with 48 cases. *Surg Neurol*. 2007;68:632–638.
33. Grant FC, Norcross NC. Repair of cranial defects by cranioplasty. *Ann Surg*. 1939;110: 488–512.
34. Brain Trauma Foundation, American Association of Neurological Surgeons, Congress of Neurological Surgeons, et al. Guidelines for the management of severe traumatic brain injury. XIII. Antiseizure prophylaxis. *J Neurotrauma*. 2007;24(suppl 1):S83–86.
35. Connolly ES Jr, Rabinstein AA, Carhuapoma JR, et al. Guidelines for the management of aneurysmal subarachnoid hemorrhage: a guideline for healthcare professionals from the American Heart Association/American Stroke Association. *Stroke*. 2012;43:1711–1737.

36. Choudhari KA, Kaliaperumal C. Three-day phenytoin prophylaxis is adequate after subarachnoid hemorrhage. *Neurosurgery*. 2007;61(author reply E):E1340.

37. Brain Trauma Foundation, American Association of Neurological Surgeons, Congress of Neurological Surgeons, et al. Guidelines for the management of severe traumatic brain injury. XII. Nutrition. *J Neurotrauma*. 2007;24(suppl 1):S77–82.

38. Guo S, Dipietro LA. Factors affecting wound healing. *J Dent Res*. 2010;89:219–229.

8

The Multicompartment Management of Intracranial Hypertension

Margaret H. Lauerman
Deborah Stein

COMPARTMENT SYNDROME AND INTRACRANIAL PRESSURE

The brain is no longer considered an isolated organ system; rather, the central nervous system (CNS) exists in a series of interconnected compartments within the body. Much as we know that therapies targeted toward intracranial pathology can affect other organ systems, therapies for and pathology in other organ systems affect the CNS. Conditions once thought benign, such as ileus, can increase intracranial pressure (ICP). We know that nursing maneuvers as simple as the height of the head of the bed can drastically change ICP. The neurointensivist must optimize all organs systems while keeping the effects of ICP in mind.

Multiple compartment syndrome (MCS) is a recently described phenomenon in which elevated pressure in extracranial body compartments, such as the thorax and the abdomen, can elevate ICP (1). MCS was described in trauma patients, where we observed that abdominal compartment syndrome (ACS) and elevated ICP often coexisted. Using a decompressive laparotomy to release the ACS also lowered ICP, even when no intervention targeted ICP. How is it that a laparotomy, which is just an incision through the skin and fascia of the abdominal wall, decreases ICP?

In order to reduce ICP, interventions that do not involve the brain may often be needed, and the neurointensivist must think outside the cranial vault.

Traditional management techniques for intracranial hypertension, such as hyperosmolar therapy with mannitol or hypertonic saline, barbiturate coma, sedation, pain control, temperature control, and induced hypothermia, may not address its underlying cause, which could lie outside the CNS in the cardiac, thoracic, or abdominal systems. These conventional ICP therapies target the volume of brain tissue, intracranial blood, and cerebrospinal fluid, and a single-minded focus on the neurologic system may miss the extracranial pathology requiring treatment in order to address ICP elevation. Therapies such as continuous renal replacement therapy (CRRT), extracorporeal membrane oxygenation (ECMO), positional therapy, and laparotomy, whose primary indications are not for ICP elevation, may actually have a therapeutic effect on elevated ICP.

However, the maximal treatment of intracranial pathology should not be forgotten, and medical and neurosurgical operative therapies should always be optimized. Patients with intracranial hypertension due to MCS often require decompressive craniectomy in addition to decompressive laparotomy. In trauma patients, decompressive craniectomy remains a prominent part of management at our institution despite recent controversy surrounding its use and its questionable mortality benefit (2). We utilize decompressive craniectomy in patients with intractable intracranial hypertension after maximal medical therapy fails.

Intrathoracic Pressure

Multiple mechanisms allow elevated intrathoracic pressure to increase ICP, including raising intracerebral arterial and venous blood volume. Intracranial venous volume increases when elevated intrathoracic pressure reduces cardiac venous return and is transmitted up through the internal jugular veins from the chest to the cranial vault (3). Normally, the cerebral venous outflow drains through a pressure gradient between the cranial vault and the thoracic cavity. This gradient lessens with elevated intrathoracic pressure. Intracranial arterial blood volume increases when elevated intrathoracic pressure reduces cardiac output because the resulting decrease in cerebral blood flow (CBF) induces compensatory cerebral arterial vasodilation.

In humans, a relationship between elevated intrathoracic pressure and intracranial hypertension has not been consistently demonstrated. Positive end-expiratory pressure (PEEP) has been used as one surrogate marker for intrathoracic pressure in lieu of direct measurement or esophageal probe measurement. However, PEEP has been shown to both increase and decrease ICP (4,5). In fact, one review found a sequential decrease in ICP with increasing levels of PEEP (4), the opposite of what would be expected if elevated intrathoracic pressure truly obstructs cranial venous outflow and lessens cardiac output (CO). One must also consider that the application of PEEP in a patient with respiratory insufficiency may improve intrathoracic compliance, which would be expected to result in improved cerebral venous return over baseline, making PEEP a poor surrogate for intrathoracic pressure. The most compelling evidence for a positive association between ICP and intrathoracic pressure was shown in an animal model, where ICP increases were seen with chest compressions (6), which should drastically increase intrathoracic pressure.

In our institution we have seen multiple cases of MCS in which elevated ICP resolves immediately with decompression of the abdomen. Although the exact pathophysiology of MCS is unknown, it seems reasonable that the effect of intraabdominal pressure on ICP is due to pressure from the abdominal cavity being transmitted to the thoracic cavity, where a column of pressure forms from the abdomen up to the cranial vault. This column of pressure would include an elevated pressure within the thoracic cavity. By this logic, elevated intrathoracic pressure without elevated intraabdominal pressure should also increase ICP. In one review looking at the effect of intraabdominal pressure on ICP, performing a sternotomy negated the ability of intraabdominal pressure to increase ICP (7) because it interrupted the column of pressure from the abdominal cavity through the thoracic cavity.

We believe that minimizing intrathoracic pressure is a sensible strategy in the management of elevated ICP. Clinically, the most common cause of elevated intrathoracic pressure is positive pressure ventilation. No enteral organs within the chest have the significant potential to distend as do those in the abdomen, and hopefully all pneumothoraces and hemothoraces will have been identified and addressed. Significant hemothoraces or pneumothoraces would exert mass effect within the thoracic cavity and can increase the plateau pressure, another potential marker of intrathoracic pressure.

Sedation and pain control, which are often used to manage ICP, have the added benefit of potentially reducing intrathoracic pressure. Increased chest wall compliance likely decreases intrathoracic pressure. Thus, propofol, benzodiazepines, and opiates, in addition to providing sedation for ICP control, will improve chest wall compliance and decrease intrathoracic pressure, which may also improve ICP through its effect on the thoracic cavity.

Ventilator strategies

Clinically, we observe that elevated intrathoracic pressure can adversely affect ICP and typically will alter our ventilator parameters to a low ventilator pressure, with low PEEP and low inspiratory pressures if clinically possible. In patients with isolated intracranial pathology without hypoxia or hypercarbia, ventilator pressures can usually be kept to minimal settings. However, in patients with concurrent pulmonary pathology that may alter lung compliance, higher ventilator pressures are often needed to maintain oxygenation. The practitioner must then balance the effects of hypoxia on inducing secondary brain injury with the possibility that increased intrathoracic pressure will reduce cranial venous outflow and decide which is more deleterious to the brain.

However, critical care practices have changed with the wide use of ARDS-net ventilation (8), and high-pressure, low-volume ventilator settings are now preferred instead of high-volume modes. Although ARDSnet ventilation is the recommended way to ventilate patients with acute respiratory distress syndrome (ARDS), it is not the only way to treat a patient with acute respiratory failure. It is common in our institution, for example, to have peak airway pressures as high as 36 mmHg on airway pressure release ventilation (APRV), which we have used in a number of patients with severe traumatic brain injury (TBI) without deleterious effects. High ventilator pressures can be required to combat concurrent pulmonary contusions, severe atelectasis, ARDS, or pulmonary edema (4). Whether this increase in ventilator pressure directly affects ICP is unknown. However, patients with TBI who have high tidal volume ventilation develop more acute lung injury (9), so a high-pressure strategy as opposed to a high-volume strategy may be most beneficial.

The optimal ventilator management strategy for patients with elevated ICP is unknown. However, when patients with TBI develop acute lung injury, they have worse outcomes (10). At our institution, patients with isolated intracranial hypertension are typically placed on volume control via synchronized intermittent mandatory ventilation (VC/SIMV) with a PEEP of 5 mmHg, an FIO_2 of 30% to 40%, and a tidal volume of 4 to 6 mL/kg in a lung protective strategy. This basic, low-pressure ventilator setting should adequately oxygenate and ventilate most patients with intracranial hypertension while assuring low intrathoracic pressure. Peak inspiratory pressure should be monitored as a surrogate of intrathoracic pressure. Hypercarbia can be addressed by increasing the minute ventilation, which should not adversely affect intrathoracic pressure.

In patients with pulmonary pathology, ventilator strategy is more difficult, as both pulmonary and intracranial pathophysiology must be considered. Ventilator settings are optimized to prevent hypoxemia, with the understanding that a concurrent increase in intrathoracic pressure may occur. With hypoxia, we will first increase the SIMV settings. Should increasing the SIMV settings fail to resolve the hypoxia, we will change ventilator modes rather than further increasing the settings on VC/SIMV. APRV is our rescue ventilator mode of choice for hypoxic patients given the constant alveolar recruitment, with an understanding that APRV likely induces a higher intrathoracic pressure than traditional ventilator modes (11).

The difference in intrathoracic pressure between ventilator modes may not be trivial, although this is similarly unknown. With SIMV, the inspiratory time usually comprises a small fraction of the respiratory cycle and depends on the inspiratory to expiratory ratio setting. Usual inspiratory to expiratory ratios in VC/SIMV range from 1:2 to 1:4, meaning that the higher intrathoracic pressures associated with inspiration in positive-pressure ventilation only occur for 20% to 33% of the respiratory cycle, with a baseline pressure of the PEEP for the remainder.

At the other extreme is APRV, in which the inspiratory to expiratory ratio is inverted. Depending on the high time (inspiratory time) and the low time (expiratory time), expiration in APRV can comprise as little as 10% of the respiratory cycle or less. The higher inspiratory pressure is then present for the majority of the respiratory cycle. Despite the physiologic effects of APRV (or other high-pressure inverse ratio modes)—with the potential for increasing intrathoracic pressure to increase ICP—neither APRV nor inverse ratio ventilation has been shown to increase ICP (12,13). In fact, patients on APRV have higher cerebral perfusion pressure (CPP) and CBF (13,14), indicating that cerebral perfusion is actually augmented.

Recruitment maneuvers are often performed in addition to conventional ventilation modes in hypoxic patients. These are set as "30 for 30" or "40 for 40," at which an inspiratory pressure of 30 or 40 mmHg is held for 30 or 40 seconds to rerecruit collapsed alveoli and improve oxygenation. These recruitment maneuvers do increase ICP, but the ICP elevation resolves when the recruitment maneuver is completed (15), assuming normal intracranial compliance.

We do not often use recruitment maneuvers at our institution, as patients either have adequate oxygenation on SIMV or are transitioned to an "open lung" ventilator strategy if hypoxic, usually with APRV. Given that open lung ventilator strategies are by definition recruitment modes of ventilation, where high, constant driving pressures are used to rerecruit collapsed alveoli, using a recruitment maneuver on top of an open lung ventilator strategy would not be beneficial. Additionally, it is unclear whether recruitment maneuvers are truly safe in patients with intracranial hypertension, given that they do induce a spike in ICP. We favor avoiding recruitment maneuvers because transient ICP elevations can be deleterious in patients with poor intracranial compliance (16).

Pressure-control ventilation (PCV) can also be used in hypoxic patients. In this ventilator mode, the PEEP is set first and then an inspiratory pressure is added on top. The inspiratory to expiratory ratio can be altered as needed for oxygenation and ventilation. Intrathoracic pressure is typically higher with this mode of ventilation than with volume control modes, given the higher driving pressures. The intrathoracic pressure in PCV is reflected by a sum of the PEEP and the inspiratory pressure, with the inspiratory time often set to a longer period when used to treat hypoxemia in a similar fashion to APRV.

For multiple reasons, we favor maximizing ventilator support as needed for hypoxia rather than allowing hypoxia through inadequate ventilation. Foremost, the data on the effect of intrathoracic pressure on ICP are less compelling than the data that hypoxia worsens neurologic outcomes. Second, should the higher intrathoracic pressure affect ICP, other pulmonary therapies, such as ECMO, prone positioning, or even a standing position (discussion to come), can improve oxygenation without high-pressure ventilation.

Jugular Venous Obstruction

In the same way that elevated intrathoracic pressure may induce intracranial hypertension, jugular venous compression is thought to increase ICP by impeding the venous outflow of the brain. Venous drainage from the cranial vault occurs through a network of veins, including the superior and inferior sagittal sinuses, straight sinus, transverse sinus, and sigmoid sinus. This venous outflow is often associated with anatomic variants at the torcular herophili, where these outflow veins converge, leaving portions of the cranial vault without the usual drainage pattern. The transverse sinus can be completely absent. The superior sagittal sinus can drain to one side and the straight sinus to the contralateral side without a central confluence of the transverse sinuses, a situation in which obstruction of either jugular vein could completely obstruct a portion of the cranial vault outflow (17). Although venous evaluation through magnetic resonance venography (MRV) does not need to be performed in all patients, neurocritical care practitioners should recognize that intracranial venous outflow may be side dominant, and unilateral jugular obstruction has the potential to completely obstruct cranial vault venous outflow given the frequency of anatomic variations. The cranial vault outflow can have collaterals outside the internal jugular vein, but this should not be relied upon in all patients (18).

Improper head positioning can obstruct the internal jugular vein. With turning of the head to either side, the ipsilateral internal jugular vein becomes narrowed on venography. With enough rotation, the vein becomes almost completely obstructed (18). Proper nursing care of patients with intracranial hypertension or at risk of elevated ICP includes maneuvers to limit internal jugular vein compression and keep the patient's head looking forward in a neutral position.

A significant number of patients with elevated ICP from TBI have concurrent cervical spine injuries requiring cervical collar immobilization. Much as twisting of the neck limits internal jugular vein flow, so does external compression, such as from a poorly fitting cervical collar. Another integral part of nursing evaluation is ensuring that the cervical collar is not compressing the neck, either globally or at a focal point. Removing the collar as early as clinically possible can limit the possibility of internal jugular vein compression. At our institution, we assess daily, after a clinical exam, whether we can remove the patient's collar. If the patient remains obtunded and unexaminable, we will obtain an MRI to radiographically confirm the absence of ligamentous injury. We will assess collar fit if long-term cervical collar use is needed, switching collar sizes (eg, to a pediatric collar for small-stature individuals) as needed for better fit or changing to Aspen® collars, as indicated.

Much like the cervical collar, other external objects can provide a similar mechanism of venous outflow obstruction. We remove all necklaces early in the hospital course. Care must be taken with endotracheal tube ties, which can compress the internal jugular vein. Similarly, tracheostomy tube ties should be assessed to ensure they are not too tight. We have seen cases of head and neck swelling from venous outflow obstruction due to tight tracheostomy ties, so this is a real clinical concern.

Patients with elevated ICP often require central venous access for medication administration, parenteral nutrition, or central venous pressure (CVP) monitoring. Traditionally, we have not placed central lines into the internal jugular vein given the concern about obstructing cerebral venous outflow as well as the increased risk of infectious complications. The potential harm to the patient with elevated ICP with internal jugular vein central line placement is twofold, with potential danger both at the time of central line placement and with chronic usage of the central line.

Both internal jugular and subclavian central line placements require the patient to tolerate the Trendelenburg position, which is used to limit the risk of venous air embolus at the time of line placement. We have seen patients with elevated ICP placed in the Trendelenburg and experience an acute elevation in ICP with just the positioning and no intervention. Thus, the decision for central access should be made with care, as positioning can certainly affect ICP. The venous cannulation itself does not seem to elevate ICP, as patients with ICP monitors do not show changes to CPP or ICP during line placement (19).

Internal jugular vein central lines can be associated with venous thrombosis. Thrombosis of the internal jugular vein has been linked with elevated ICP in multiple case reports (20). Thus, patients with elevated ICP should have either subclavian or femoral central lines placed should large-bore intravenous access be required. In emergency situations, such as with hypotension, we will place a femoral line for immediate access. However, in a stable patient, we will place a subclavian central line preferentially to avoid the risk of internal jugular vein obstruction, assuming that the patient can tolerate positioning for placement without ICP elevation.

There is also a possibility that thrombosis in the internal jugular vein can propagate back to the intracranial veins. In the International Study on Cerebral Vein and Dural Sinus Thrombosis (ISCVT), while the most common inciting factors of intracranial venous thrombosis included hematologic abnormalities, pregnancy, and malignancy, the inciting factor in multiple patients was internal jugular catheter placement (21).

Supine and Prone Positioning

Patient posture is an important consideration in the care of patients with intracranial pathology. Small changes in the angle of the head of the bed can make large differences in intracerebral hemodynamics. In stroke patients, there is a stepwise association with head positioning, ICP, and cerebral hemodynamics. Laying the patient at 15 degrees of head elevation compared to 30 degrees produces an increase in ICP and a concurrent increase in mean arterial pressure (MAP) and CPP. The changes in MAP, CPP, and ICP continue in a similar fashion when the patient is placed completely supine compared with a 15-degree or 30-degree elevation of the head of the bed (22).

The effects of posture on ICP seen in stroke patients is similarly seen in patients with TBI. In patients with TBI, supine positioning is associated with an increase in ICP, and ICP measurements are often above 20 mmHg. However, in contrast to patients with strokes, supine positioning is not associated with a change in CPP or CBF. Patients with normal ICP seem to be less affected by the supine position than patients with elevated ICP (23).

Given that head elevation is associated with a lower ICP without concurrent changes in CPP or CBF, we elevate the head of the bed greater than 30 degrees in all patients with elevated ICP as a cerebroprotective strategy. At our institution, almost all patients with intracranial hypertension can be positioned with their head elevated rather than supine, including those patients in traction for femur or acetabular fractures, those in external fixation for pelvic fractures, and those with open abdomens. Patients with spine fractures are evaluated for early fixation or bracing to facilitate mobilization. In patients who must lie flat due to spinal fractures, we will place the bed in a reverse Trendelenburg to elevate the head while keeping the spine in a neutral position. No patients with elevated ICP should be left supine. However, positioning does not seem to have as much of an effect on patients with intracranial pathology but no elevated ICP.

Elevating the head of the bed is not the only positioning consideration in the critically ill patient. Prone positioning is used for patients with respiratory failure and has recently been validated as improving outcomes in acute respiratory failure. In a randomized multicenter trial, prone positioning for ARDS was associated with a 16.8% absolute reduction in mortality at 28 days (24). Prone positioning should be considered in all patients with refractory hypoxemia or severe respiratory failure and is the penultimate maneuver in our institution for hypoxic respiratory failure prior to extracorporeal membrane oxygenation (ECMO) cannulation.

We utilize increasing ventilator pressures and rescue modes of ventilation, including APRV and PCV, prior to using prone positioning. In patients with severe refractory hypoxemia or hypercarbia, we often initiate ECMO and prone positioning simultaneously. Prone positioning is thought to be especially beneficial in patients with posterior pulmonary collapse, which can be off-loaded and allowed to rerecruit in the prone position.

Prone positioning can be accomplished in multiple ways. The simplest is by moving the patient from one bed to another or turning the patient within his or her own bed, although this can be difficult in the obese. Prone positioning frames, where the patient can be secured into place on the frame and rotated into the prone position, are available. When using prone positioning, care must be taken to pad pressure points, as skin breakdown can occur, most often on the forehead and the chin. Prone positioning should only be initiated with an experienced medical team, including multiple nurses and physicians present at the bedside, as the potential exists for rapid respiratory decompensation when the patient is initially placed prone. The severity of the respiratory failure and how well the patient responds to prone or supine positioning determines its duration, although we generally keep the patient prone for 4 to 8 hours, or longer if the patient's oxygenation responds well.

Despite its well-proven benefits on oxygenation, prone positioning may be harmful to patients with elevated ICP. In one study, a majority of patients with intracranial pathology had an elevation in ICP when placed prone. When these patients were changed from the supine to the prone position, there was a 5.9 mmHg mean increase in ICP and a concurrent 7.9 mmHg mean decrease in MAP, and more episodes of low CPP were recorded while patients were prone (25).

The risks and benefits must be carefully evaluated in patients with intracranial pathology prior to prone positioning. Patients with ICP monitors but without elevated ICP may still be candidates for prone positioning. In contrast, given the increase in ICP seen with prone positioning, patients with elevated ICP may not be ideal candidates but instead should be considered for standing positioning or ECMO if they have failed conventional and rescue modes of ventilation. Alternatively, if prone positioning markedly improves intrathoracic compliance, its beneficial effect on intrathoracic pressure and oxygenation may offset its detriment on ICP. In this situation, clinical judgment must be applied. In some cases, the harm of increasing ICP outweighs the benefits of improved oxygenation while prone, and improved oxygenation can also be achieved through ECMO or standing positioning without the concurrent increase in ICP.

Standing Positioning

Patients with baseline elevated ICP and severe respiratory failure are difficult to treat. Increasing the driving pressure for ventilation may increase intrathoracic pressure and thus ICP. Using the prone position may be associated with increased ICP, as well. ECMO may be helpful in some patients with elevated ICP but is not widely available. At our institution, for patients with refractory hypoxemia and TBI, we favor standing positioning and/or ECMO use. The standing position allows for recruitment of the posterior pulmonary segments, as does the prone position, without the increased ICP seen in patients in the prone position. The physiologic rationale for standing is the same as for prone positioning—off-loading of the posterior pulmonary segments to allow rerecruitment and improve oxygenation.

To stand a patient, a specialized board is needed. The board requires a footrest to stabilize the patient as well as straps to hold the patient securely in place. The only limitations to standing patients are orthopedic, as we have used the standing position in patients with concurrent open abdomens and ECMO cannulation. Patients do need sedation and/or paralysis, although this is often already being used for intracranial hypertension. Standing positioning requires an experienced nursing staff to assure patient safety and should only be undertaken in experienced centers with the proper equipment.

Aside from being an excellent tool for pulmonary recruitment in patients with elevated ICP and hypoxia, the standing position may benefit patients with refractory intracranial hypertension without respiratory failure. ICP has been shown to decrease in patients in the standing position when compared with the supine position, although these patients did not have elevated ICP at baseline (26). In some cases, ICP decreased sequentially when the patient was moved from supine to sitting to standing (27).

Unfortunately, there is little guidance in the literature as to the benefit of standing positioning. Although we do use the standing position in our patients, it is mostly limited to those with concurrent respiratory failure who would need prone positioning, which their concurrent TBI may contraindicate. Standing positioning is not specifically stated as a primary strategy in our protocol for elevated ICP. Rather, we favor strategies such as maximizing hyperosmolar therapy and decompressive craniectomy. The evidence for standing positioning is sparse, and the risk to the patient is not trivial.

Systemic Hypoxia

Hypoxia can stem from a variety of pulmonary causes in patients with elevated ICP. Patients with TBI often have concurrent pulmonary contusions, hemothoraces, or pneumothoraces that can induce hypoxia. Patients in the intensive care unit (ICU) can also have pulmonary edema, ARDS, or pneumonia. Despite ventilator manipulation or patient positioning, hypoxia may be persistent.

Systemic hypoxia can increase ICP, an effect that is mediated through CBF (28). When a patient is normoxemic, CBF does not change with varying arterial oxygen pressure (PaO_2) levels. Starting at a PaO_2 of approximately 53 mmHg, CBF begins to increase as hypoxia worsens. This increase in CBF with hypoxia is not minimal; for example, when the PaO_2 falls from 50 to 25 mmHg, the CBF doubles (29).

Although this increasing CBF is usually a protective measure to assure cerebral oxygenation in the setting of systemic hypoxia, in patients with intracranial hypertension, elevations in CBF can be harmful. The increase in CBF is not just an increase in blood flow velocity or volume of blood flow; rather, the increase in CBF occurs due to cerebral vasodilation (28). Intracranial vasodilation will increase the intracranial volume, leading to an increase in ICP as the space within the cranial vault is restricted by the skull and cannot expand.

Given the association between hypoxia and cerebral vasodilation, it is not surprising that systemic hypoxia is an independent predictor of outcomes following TBI (30). Despite the compensatory increase in CBF seen with systemic hypoxia, lower brain oxygenation is observed in patients with higher ICP (31). Hyperoxia is also associated with worse outcomes (32), and the ideal oxygenation level for patients with elevated ICP remains unknown.

At our institution, we follow the same oxygenation parameters in patients with elevated ICP that we do for all other critically ill patients. We keep the fraction of inspired oxygen (FIO_2) at a level that permits adequate oxygen saturation but avoids hyperoxia. We do not routinely monitor PaO_2, however, as an adequate oxygen saturation is above the PaO_2 level at which CBF increases.

The role of extracorporeal membrane oxygenation

EMCO is a support maneuver of last resort in patients with severe pulmonary dysfunction, either with hypoxemia or hypercarbia. Although the randomized controlled Conventional Ventilation or ECMO for Severe Adult Respiratory Failure (CESAR) trial did not ultimately show a significant benefit to ECMO use in respiratory failure (33), we have successfully used ECMO at our institution to bridge patients with respiratory failure who had failed conventional ventilation maneuvers. At this point, ECMO is only available in select tertiary care centers.

ECMO enables support either with veno-venous bypass (VV) or arterio-venous bypass (VA). In general, patients with isolated respiratory failure are supported with VV-ECMO because it requires only venous cannulation. Cannulation is usually accomplished through the internal jugular vein and femoral vein, the femoral vein bilaterally, or by using an Avalon Elite® single-lumen catheter inserted through the internal jugular vein. In patients with elevated ICP, femoral vein cannulation is preferred given the large-bore access needed and the potential for internal jugular vein obstruction with this access. VA-ECMO is reserved for patients with concurrent cardiac dysfunction. VA-ECMO would not be required in patients with elevated ICP and may be contraindicated due to the absolute requirement for systemic anticoagulation.

In a hypoxemic patient with elevated ICP, correcting the hypoxemia is paramount to limiting secondary brain injury. When ECMO is initiated, systemic oxygenation usually improves. Whether cerebral perfusion parameters improve is less clear. The intracranial physiology is more complicated, as it involves interplay with CO_2 levels and cerebral autoregulation.

One patient without intracranial pathology whose cerebral oxygenation was monitored while on ECMO showed improved systemic oxygenation but a decrease in cerebral oxygenation as systemic CO_2 decreased. It is thought that improved CO_2 clearance after ECMO initiation increases the pH, which in turn may move the oxygen dissociation curve. This may decrease cerebral oxygen delivery despite increasing systemic oxygenation with ECMO (34). Additionally, the lower CO_2 seen in patients placed on ECMO may result in reflexive cerebral vasoconstriction and a reduction in CBF, much as hyperventilation does.

In the same case, MAP also declined after starting ECMO, which decreased the CPP in the setting of elevated ICP. Although patients without intracranial pathology should autoregulate CBF, when autoregulation is lost, a decrease in MAP may significantly decrease CBF (34). The use of near-infrared spectroscopy (NIRS), a marker of intracerebral perfusion, showed a direct correlation between CO_2 levels and CBF (35). Fortunately for patients with respiratory failure who require ECMO and have a concurrently elevated ICP, good outcomes for ECMO patients are correlated with a small decrease in CO_2 after the initiation of ECMO (36).

The use of ECMO, aside from its beneficial effect on oxygenation, may also decrease ICP, much as the use of CRRT may decrease ICP. In animals and humans, ICP decreased after ECMO initiation and remained decreased at 48 hours (37,38). ECMO has been shown to be a feasible treatment in patients with intracranial pathology, with good short- and long-term outcomes. In one case series, seven patients with TBI who were treated with ECMO had an 86% survival rate and a median Glasgow Coma Scale (GCS) score on discharge of 14 (39). ECMO could be regarded as a potential therapeutic intervention for elevated ICP, but data are limited to small-animal studies and case series at this time.

The management of a patient with elevated ICP on ECMO can be a challenging clinical situation, as ECMO circuits are traditionally run with full systemic anticoagulation. Anticoagulation is mandatory in VA-ECMO given the concern of thrombosis on the arterial side, where clots can result in arterial thrombosis, pulmonary emboli, or stroke. In patients with TBI and elevated ICP, there are multiple ways of running ECMO to avoid the use of systemic anticoagulation, including employing heparin-bonded circuits (40) or a pumpless device (37). In patients with isolated elevation in CO_2, the NovaLung® can be used instead of ECMO (41). At our institution, we have run VV-ECMO without systemic anticoagulation when left with no other options, but we will not run VA-ECMO without systemic anticoagulation due to the devastating potential consequences of embolism.

Intraabdominal Pressure

A wide variety of conditions ranging from ileus to visceral edema to intraabdominal hemorrhage to ascites can induce an elevated intraabdominal pressure. Many patients in the ICU have elevated intraabdominal pressure, with one review reporting an incidence of 32% (42). Although some patients may present with concurrent intraabdominal and intracranial pathology, other patients will develop elevated intraabdominal pressure over the ICU course. For example, patients in the ICU can develop a secondary event such as sepsis, leading to excessive fluid resuscitation, or retroperitoneal edema from pancreatitis, conditions completely unrelated to their intracranial pathology.

An evaluation for intraabdominal hypertension (IAH) should begin with the physical exam, evaluating for a distended, tense abdomen. Bladder pressures are most commonly used to monitor for elevation in intraabdominal pressure and are easily measured at the bedside by injecting 50 mL of sterile fluid through the Foley catheter and transducing the pressure (43). For the most accurate measurement, the patient should be flat and paralyzed, although if the bladder pressure is low and the patient is not completely sedated, the true bladder pressure is probably low.

Elevated intraabdominal pressure exists at a bladder pressure over 12 mmHg (44). ACS has traditionally been defined as an intraabdominal pressure exceeding 20 mmHg when combined with end-organ dysfunction (45), such as renal failure. Despite these numerical guidelines, ACS should not be excluded in the presence of end-organ dysfunction if the bladder pressure is less than 20 mmHg, and it should always be evaluated in the appropriate clinical context.

Multiple markers of organ dysfunction can indicate ACS. Oliguria or renal failure can indicate ACS, although this measurement is invalid in patients already in renal failure, which is common in the ICU. Elevated peak airway pressures from decreased diaphragm excursion can indicate ACS; however, care should be taken to evaluate peak airway pressures while in a volume-control ventilator mode. In a PCV mode, peak airway pressures will not increase with ACS; rather, the tidal volumes will decrease with the same peak airway pressure. Hypotension can be seen due to a decreased venous return to the heart from the abdominal cavity. Ultimately, if left untreated, ACS can result in decreases in gastrointestinal, renal, and hepatic blood flow with subsequent organ failure or intestinal ischemia. If untreated, ACS can progress to multiorgan dysfunction and death (46).

Elevated intraabdominal pressure should be managed according to guidelines from the World Society of Abdominal Compartment Syndrome (47). Patients should be sedated and if necessary, chemically paralyzed. Patients should have gastric and rectal decompression. The initial treatment includes fluid removal with diuresis or dialysis, if hemodynamically tolerated. All patients should be evaluated for ascites with bedside ultrasound, a readily available tool. If ascites exists, paracentesis should be performed (44) to lessen the intraabdominal contents. A decompressive laparotomy is reserved for refractory cases.

Although only a small amount of literature examines the relationship between intraabdominal pressure and ICP, increasing intraabdominal pressure is associated with increased ICP in both humans and animal models (48,49). In fact, ICP increases sequentially as intraabdominal pressure increases (48) and is likely mediated by elevated intrathoracic pressure as elevated intraabdominal pressure decreases lung compliance, functional residual capacity (FRC), cardiac index, and CO (7,45).

Laparotomy for refractory intracranial hypertension

A decompressive laparotomy is the gold standard surgical therapy for patients with ACS. A laparotomy releases pressure in the abdomen through opening the fascia and skin, both of which can constrict the expansion of the intraabdominal contents. However, after a decompressive laparotomy, patients are exposed to the risks of an open abdomen, which include enterocutaneous fistula and renal failure (50). Repairing the ventral hernia requires another operation, which is often a complicated surgical reconstruction of the abdominal wall.

In an elective laparotomy, the fascia and the skin of the abdominal wall are closed upon completing the procedure. When a decompressive laparotomy is performed for elevated ICP, the abdominal wall is left open. The visceral organs, including the small intestine, colon, stomach, and liver, are left exposed, and the abdomen is covered with a temporary dressing, including vacuum dressings or suturing IV bags to the fascia. Ultimately, when the ACS resolves, the fascia and the skin are closed at the index admission, if possible. Otherwise, the fascia is left open, the viscera are covered with a skin graft or native skin coverage, and a planned ventral hernia repair for definitive closure is undertaken in the future.

ICP reduction after a decompressive laparotomy in patients with intracranial hypertension and elevated intraabdominal pressure has been well demonstrated. The largest series describing this intervention for intracranial hypertension comes from our institution, which examined 102 patients who required a decompressive craniectomy for elevated ICP. A decompressive laparotomy for IAH was concurrently performed in 24% of these patients. ICP decreased by an average of 9 mmHg following abdominal decompression (1).

A decompressive laparotomy can be used without a decompressive craniectomy for treating elevated ICP, as well (51,52). In our institution, we evaluate all patients with intracranial hypertension for concomitantly elevated intraabdominal pressure. We perform physical exams for evidence of abdominal distention or abdominal wall tension, and if concern exists we will transduce a bladder pressure to confirm IAH.

Patients with elevated ICP, elevated intrathoracic pressure, and elevated intraabdominal pressure are described as having MCS or polycompartment syndrome (53). Fortunately, the incidence of MCS is relatively rare and seen in only 2% of patients with TBI (1). Multicompartment pressure elevation must be taken seriously, as mortality rises to as high as 42% in patients with MCS (1,51). However, from our recent clinical experience, the incidence of MCS is decreasing due to changes in resuscitation patterns, with less crystalloid administration, permissive hypotension, and early blood product administration.

A decompressive laparotomy can be lifesaving in patients with MCS. Good functional outcome after abdominal decompression has been achieved (52), and we feel that the morbidity associated with an open abdomen is less than the morbidity of continued refractory intracranial hypertension. We will consider a decompressive laparotomy on patients with elevated intraabdominal pressure and intractable intracranial hypertension. There is a benefit to earlier decompressive laparotomy (51), so we evaluate patients early and often for MCS. The order in which decompressive laparotomy and decompressive craniectomy are undertaken does not seem to influence outcomes (1).

Volume Status

Resuscitation patterns in critical care have drastically changed over the last decade. In the past, we would give many liters of crystalloid during resuscitation, with resultant pulmonary edema, visceral edema, and anasarca. We focus now on goal-directed resuscitation, the more liberal use of vasoconstrictors, and using markers of resuscitation to guide fluid or blood administration because we know that liberal use of fluid is detrimental (54). Markers such as lactate, base excess, stroke volume variation (SVV), and CVP are used to provide end points of resuscitation. Hypotension is more tolerated in the modern era.

However, we know there is potential harm from hypovolemia in patients with intracranial pathology, putting resuscitation of the patient with elevated ICP at odds with current resuscitation strategies. A negative fluid balance is an independent predictor of poor neurologic outcome in patients with brain injury, and patients with a negative fluid balance necessitate more ICP therapy with mannitol (55).

Additionally, systemic hypotension causes secondary brain injury through intracranial hypoperfusion. A decrease in CPP due to systemic hypovolemia may be heightened in patients with elevated ICP, in which an adequate CPP relies on maintaining a higher MAP to counteract the elevated ICP. A historical dictum in managing patients with elevated ICP states that hypovolemia decreases cerebral edema; however, this practice is not currently supported (55) given what we understand about the maintenance of cerebral perfusion.

Although we know that hypovolemia is not optimal for patients with elevated ICP, their optimal volume status remains unknown. In trauma patients with TBI, fluid is often given to support systemic blood pressure, which may be decreased due to concurrent injuries, such as hemorrhage or spinal cord injury. Fluid may be given in general to patients with intracranial hypertension to support a MAP or CPP goal. Critically ill patients are much more likely to be hypervolemic than hypovolemic or even euvolemic, however, and data suggest that TBI patients who receive more fluids have worse outcomes (56,57). Unfortunately, both hypovolemia and hypervolemia appear to be harmful in brain injury.

We have seen a decrease in MCS at our institution with the decrease in massive crystalloid resuscitation. Fluid resuscitation volumes likely play a significant role in the development of elevated ICP in MCS. Patients who ultimately required a decompressive laparotomy for IAH and ICP elevation had received an additional 23 liters of fluid when compared with patients who did not require a decompressive laparotomy, and ascites was almost universally seen in these patients at the time of the laparotomy (1). Fluid administration, although necessary in some patients to support CPP, produces visceral and abdominal wall edema and likely plays a large role in inducing MCS.

Although the optimal fluid balance remains to be elucidated, the management of volume status in patients with elevated ICP should utilize markers of resuscitation, such as a MAP greater than 65 mmHg, the normalization of lactate levels, and the maintenance of urine output at greater than 0.5 mL/kg, while maintaining CPP targets (58).

At our institution, we commonly use 3% saline to resuscitate patients with elevated ICP because it acts as both a volume expander and an osmotic therapy (59). We avoid albumin because the Saline vs. Albumin Fluid Evaluation (SAFE) trial consistently showed an increase in mortality in TBI patients receiving it (60). Otherwise, we favor the judicious use of normal saline with careful monitoring of CPP, MAP, and urine output.

We use multiple modalities of measuring volume status in our ICUs. Noninvasive Flo Trac Vigileo™ (Edwards Lifesciences Corporation) monitoring is used to measure CO and SVV using an arterial line tracing (61). Pulmonary artery catheters are rarely used and only in patients with known cardiac dysfunction. Echocardiography, through use of the focused rapid echocardiographic examination (FREE), provides a bedside evaluation of volume status and is often used to guide resuscitation (62).

Renal Failure

Acute renal failure (ARF) occurs in 30% of hospitalized patients in the ICU (63). Although the exact incidence in patients with intracranial hypertension is unknown, several studies of patients with intracranial pathology (e.g., stroke, subarachnoid hemorrhage) demonstrated an incidence of acute kidney injury (AKI) of 23% to 27% (64,65). In patients with TBI, the incidence is thought to be around 10% (66). Patients who progress to ARF may indicate a need for renal replacement therapy.

The main issue concerning renal replacement therapy (RRT) and ICP elevation in patients with acute or chronic kidney injury is how to safely dialyze and remove excess volume. Another issue is whether CRRT has a secondary benefit of reducing ICP beyond its known indications of addressing electrolyte imbalances, uremia, and hypervolemia.

Multiple methods of volume management can be used for patients with intracranial hypertension. The options available for removing fluid in patients with oliguric or anuric renal failure are intermittent hemodialysis (IHD) or CRRT. In ICU patients, IHD is commonly used in hemodynamically stable patients, and CRRT is used in hemodynamically unstable patients who cannot tolerate the rapid fluid shifts associated with IHD. However, there are concerns about IHD safety in patients with ICP elevation, and IHD may never be an appropriate option in intracranial hypertension. IHD has been reported to increase ICP and decrease CPP, changes that are not seen with CRRT (67). The complications of IHD in elevated ICP were not limited to changes in intracranial perfusion, as one case series reported an 80% mortality rate with IHD use in patients with intracranial hemorrhage (68).

IHD decreases osmolality (67) and urea gradient (69), which contributes to cerebral edema and increases ICP. There may be ways of altering the IHD parameters to make the IHD runs safer in patients with intracranial pathology (70). The goals of these modified IHD parameters include avoiding hypotension at the initiation of IHD and during the IHD run, preventing decreases in CPP, and minimizing osmolality shifts. Practical strategies for IHD in patients with intracranial hypertension include planning shorter-duration IHD sessions and using smaller dialyzers to reduce the speed of urea removal. IHD can be scheduled more frequently, instead of the usual three times weekly, lessening the urea shift during each IHD session. This may induce less cerebral edema. Lower bicarbonate solutions can also be used to minimize paradoxical intracellular acidosis (69).

Practically, CRRT has advantages over IHD beyond the traditional indications for dialysis. Patients on CRRT can have fluid removed as needed, while patients treated with IHD are limited to fluid removal during the dialysis session, often requiring fluid and protein restriction. In an ICU patient, this can mean limiting nutritional intake. This restriction is unnecessary for patients on CRRT.

CRRT may also benefit those with intracranial hypertension beyond its traditional indications of fluid removal and dialysis. CRRT has been reported to decrease ICP in cases of refractory intracranial hypertension. In one review of four patients with elevated ICP who were on CRRT, three had improved ICP after the initiation of CRRT. This decrease in ICP occurred within hours of CRRT initiation and, given the rapidity of the drop, was not likely due to volume removal alone (71).

CRRT has even been used for the sole purpose of decreasing ICP in a patient with refractory intracranial hypertension without renal failure. In this patient, ICP dropped immediately after the initiation of CRRT with the removal of only a small amount of fluid. Although the true mechanism is unknown, the rapid drop in ICP after beginning CRRT may be due to cytokine removal (72). In addition to possible beneficial effects with respect to inflammatory mediator removal, the maintenance of normothermia and relative hypernatremia are other potential mechanisms of improved ICP control in patients on CRRT (73).

At our institution, we start critically ill patients with oliguric or anuric renal failure on CRRT. This allows us to carefully titrate volume status, electrolytes, and acid-base status. IHD is only used in stable chronically ill patients. In patients with intracranial hypertension refractory to medical therapy, we aggressively maximize medical therapy and pursue a decompressive craniectomy, if needed. CRRT is not currently considered a primary therapy for intractable ICP elevation in the absence of renal failure at our institution, and we would caution that more research needs to be done before recommending CRRT as a primary modality for ICP management.

CONCLUSIONS

The control of elevated ICP cannot focus solely on therapies within the cranial vault, as pressures within other body compartments can affect ICP as well. Ventilators must be set to limit intrathoracic pressure and hypoxia. Patient positioning should allow optimal venous outflow from the cranial vault. Attention should be paid to volume resuscitation strategies and identifying IAH. Adjunctive therapies, such as CRRT and standing positioning, should be considered in elevated ICP. ECMO seems to be a safe treatment for refractory hypoxia with intracranial hypertension. Future research will delineate the optimal care of the patient with elevated ICP when considering all body compartments.

References

1. Scalea TM, Bochicchio GV, Habashi N, et al. Increased intra-abdominal, intrathoracic, and intracranial pressure after severe brain injury: multiple compartment syndrome. *J Trauma*. 2007;62(3):647–656;(discussion):656.

2. Cooper DJ, Rosenfeld JV, Murray L, et al. Decompressive craniectomy in diffuse traumatic brain injury. *N Engl J Med*. 2011;364(16):1493–1502.

3. Ngubane T. Mechanical ventilation and the injured brain. *Southern African Journal of Anaesthesia and Analgesia*. 2014;17(1):76–80.

4. Huynh T, Messer M, Sing RF, et al. Positive end-expiratory pressure alters intracranial and cerebral perfusion pressure in severe traumatic brain injury. *J Trauma*. 2002;53(3): 488–92;(discussion):492–493.

5. Cooper KR, Boswell PA, Choi SC. Safe use of PEEP in patients with severe head injury. *J Neurosurg*. 1985;63(4):552–555.

6. Guerci AD, Shi AY, Levin H, et al. Transmission of intrathoracic pressure to the intracranial space during cardiopulmonary resuscitation in dogs. *Circ Res*. 1985;56(1):20–30.

7. Bloomfield GL, Ridings PC, Blocher CR, et al. A proposed relationship between increased intra-abdominal, intrathoracic, and intracranial pressure. *Crit Care Med*. 1997; 25(3):496–503.

8. Acute Respiratory Distress Syndrome Network. Ventilation with lower tidal volumes as compared with traditional tidal volumes for acute lung injury and the acute respiratory distress syndrome. *N Engl J Med*. 2000;342(18):1301–1308.

9. Mascia L, Zavala E, Bosma K, et al. High tidal volume is associated with the development of acute lung injury after severe brain injury: an international observational study. *Crit Care Med*. 2007;35(8):1815–1820.

10. Holland MC, Mackersie RC, Morabito D, et al. The development of acute lung injury is associated with worse neurologic outcome in patients with severe traumatic brain injury. *J Trauma*. 2003;55(1):106–111.

11. Andrews P, Habashi N. Airway pressure release ventilation. *Curr Probl Surg*. 2013;50(10): 462–470.

12. Clarke JP. The effects of inverse ratio ventilation on intracranial pressure: a preliminary report. *Intensive Care Med*. 1997;23(1):106–109.

13. Marik PE, Young A, Sibole S, et al. The effect of APRV ventilation on ICP and cerebral hemodynamics. *Neurocrit Care*. 2012;17(2):219–223.

14. Kreyer S, Putensen C, Berg A, et al. Effects of spontaneous breathing during airway pressure release ventilation on cerebral and spinal cord perfusion in experimental acute lung injury. *J Neurosurg Anesthesiol*. 2010;22(4):323–329.

15. Zhang XY, Yang ZJ, Wang QX, et al. Impact of positive end-expiratory pressure on cerebral injury patients with hypoxemia. *Am J Emerg Med*. 2011;29(7):699–703.

16. Stein DM, Hu PF, Brenner M, et al. Brief episodes of intracranial hypertension and cerebral hypoperfusion are associated with poor functional outcome after severe traumatic brain injury. *J Trauma*. 2011;71(2):364–373;(discussion):373–374.

17. Gokce E, Pinarbasili T, Acu B, et al. Torcular herophili classification and evaluation of dural venous sinus variations using digital subtraction angiography and magnetic resonance venographies. *Surg Radiol Anat*. 2014;36(6):527–536.

18. Gooding CA, Stimac GK. Jugular vein obstruction caused by turning of the head. *AJR Am J Roentgenol.* 1984;142(2):403–406.

19. Woda RP, Miner ME, McCandless C, et al. The effect of right internal jugular vein cannulation on intracranial pressure. *J Neurosurg Anesthesiol.* 1996;8(4):286–292.

20. Duke BJ, Ryu RK, Brega KE, et al. Traumatic bilateral jugular vein thrombosis: case report and review of the literature. *Neurosurgery.* 1997;41(3):680–683.

21. Ferro JM, Canhao P, Stam J, et al. Prognosis of cerebral vein and dural sinus thrombosis: results of the International Study on Cerebral Vein and Dural Sinus Thrombosis (ISCVT). *Stroke.* 2004;35(3):664–670.

22. Schwarz S, Georgiadis D, Aschoff A, et al. Effects of body position on intracranial pressure and cerebral perfusion in patients with large hemispheric stroke. *Stroke.* 2002;33(2):497–501.

23. Feldman Z, Kanter MJ, Robertson CS, et al. Effect of head elevation on intracranial pressure, cerebral perfusion pressure, and cerebral blood flow in head-injured patients. *J Neurosurg.* 1992;76(2):207–211.

24. Guerin C, Reignier J, Richard JC, et al. Prone positioning in severe acute respiratory distress syndrome. *N Engl J Med.* 2013;368(23):2159–2168.

25. Roth C, Ferbert A, Deinsberger W, et al. Does prone positioning increase intracranial pressure? A retrospective analysis of patients with acute brain injury and acute respiratory failure. *Neurocrit Care.* 2014;21(2):186–191.

26. Andresen M, Hadi A, Petersen LG, et al. Effect of postural changes on ICP in healthy and ill subjects. *Acta Neurochir* (Vienna). 2015;157(1):109–113.

27. Andresen M, Juhler M. Intracranial pressure following complete removal of a small demarcated brain tumor: a model for normal intracranial pressure in humans. *J Neurosurg.* 2014;121(4):797–801.

28. Kety SS, Schmidt CF. The effects of altered arterial tensions of carbon dioxide and oxygen on cerebral blood flow and cerebral oxygen consumption of normal young men. *J Clin Invest.* 1948;27(4):484–492.

29. Johnston AJ, Steiner LA, Gupta AK, et al. Cerebral oxygen vasoreactivity and cerebral tissue oxygen reactivity. *Br J Anaesth.* 2003;90(6):774–786.

30. McHugh GS, Engel DC, Butcher I, et al. Prognostic value of secondary insults in traumatic brain injury: results from the IMPACT study. *J Neurotrauma.* 2007;24(2):287–293.

31. Oddo M, Levine JM, Mackenzie L, et al. Brain hypoxia is associated with short-term outcome after severe traumatic brain injury independently of intracranial hypertension and low cerebral perfusion pressure. *Neurosurgery.* 2011;69(5):1037–1045;(discussion):1045.

32. Brenner M, Stein D, Hu P, et al. Association between early hyperoxia and worse outcomes after traumatic brain injury. *Arch Surg.* 2012;147(11):1042–1046.

33. Peek GJ, Mugford M, Tiruvoipati R, et al. Efficacy and economic assessment of conventional ventilatory support versus extracorporeal membrane oxygenation for severe adult respiratory failure (CESAR): a multicentre randomised controlled trial. *Lancet.* 2009;374(9698):1351–1363.

34. Muellenbach RM, Kilgenstein C, Kranke P, et al. Effects of venovenous extracorporeal membrane oxygenation on cerebral oxygenation in hypercapnic ARDS. *Perfusion.* 2014;29(2):139–141.

35. Quarti A, Nardone S, Manfrini F, et al. Effect of the adjunct of carbon dioxide during cardiopulmonary bypass on cerebral oxygenation. *Perfusion.* 2013;28(2):152–155.

36. Bembea MM, Lee R, Masten D, et al. Magnitude of arterial carbon dioxide change at initiation of extracorporeal membrane oxygenation support is associated with survival. *J Extra Corpor Technol.* 2013;45(1):26–32.

37. Bein T, Scherer MN, Philipp A, et al. Pumpless extracorporeal lung assist (pECLA) in patients with acute respiratory distress syndrome and severe brain injury. *J Trauma.* 2005;58(6):1294–1297.

38. Liem KD, Kollee LA, Klaessens JH, et al. The influence of extracorporeal membrane oxygenation on cerebral oxygenation and hemodynamics in normoxemic and hypoxemic piglets. *Pediatr Res.* 1996;39(2):209–215.

39. Biderman P, Einav S, Fainblut M, et al. Extracorporeal life support in patients with multiple injuries and severe respiratory failure: a single-center experience? *J Trauma Acute Care Surg.* 2013;75(5):907–912.

40. Reynolds HN, Cottingham C, McCunn M, et al. Extracorporeal lung support in a patient with traumatic brain injury: the benefit of heparin-bonded circuitry. *Perfusion.* 1999;14(6):489–493.

41. Mallick A, Elliot S, McKinlay J, et al. Extracorporeal carbon dioxide removal using the Novalung in a patient with intracranial bleeding. *Anaesthesia.* 2007;62(1):72–74.

42. Malbrain ML, Chiumello D, Pelosi P, et al. Incidence and prognosis of intraabdominal hypertension in a mixed population of critically ill patients: a multiple-center epidemiological study. *Crit Care Med.* 2005;33(2):315–322.

43. Fusco MA, Martin RS, Chang MC. Estimation of intra-abdominal pressure by bladder pressure measurement: validity and methodology. *J Trauma.* 2001;50(2):297–302.

44. Kirkpatrick AW, Roberts DJ, De Waele J, et al. Intra-abdominal hypertension and the abdominal compartment syndrome: updated consensus definitions and clinical practice guidelines from the World Society of the Abdominal Compartment Syndrome. *Intensive Care Med.* 2013;39(7):1190–1206.

45. Malbrain ML, Cheatham ML. Definitions and pathophysiological implications of intra-abdominal hypertension and abdominal compartment syndrome. *Am Surg.* 2011;77(suppl 1): S–611.

46. Cheatham ML. Abdominal compartment syndrome: pathophysiology and definitions. *Scand J Trauma Resusc Emerg Med.* 2009;17:10.

47. World Society of the Abdominal Compartment Syndrome, *IAH/ACS Management Algorithm.* 2014; https://www.wsacs.org/images/algorithms/IAH_ACS_management_2014.pdf. Accessed April 3, 2015.

48. Saggi BH, Bloomfield GL, Sugerman HJ, et al. Treatment of intracranial hypertension using nonsurgical abdominal decompression. *J Trauma.* 1999;46(4):646–651.

49. Citerio G, Vascotto E, Villa F, et al. Induced abdominal compartment syndrome increases intracranial pressure in neurotrauma patients: a prospective study. *Crit Care Med.* 2001;29(7): 1466–1471.

50. Dubose JJ, Scalea TM, Holcomb JB, et al. Open abdominal management after damage-control laparotomy for trauma: a prospective observational American Association for the Surgery of Trauma multicenter study. *J Trauma Acute Care Surg.* 2013;74(1):113–120;(discussion):1120–1122.

51. Joseph DK, Dutton RP, Aarabi B, et al. Decompressive laparotomy to treat intractable intracranial hypertension after traumatic brain injury. *J Trauma.* 2004;57(4):687–693;(discussion):693–695.

52. Miglietta MA, Salzano LJ, Chiu WC, et al. Decompressive laparotomy: a novel approach in the management of severe intracranial hypertension. *J Trauma.* 2003;55(3):551–554;(discussion):554–555.

53. Malbrain ML, Wilmer A. The polycompartment syndrome: towards an understanding of the interactions between different compartments! *Intensive Care Med.* 2007;33(11):1869–1872.

54. Kasotakis G, Sideris A, Yang Y, et al. Aggressive early crystalloid resuscitation adversely affects outcomes in adult blunt trauma patients: an analysis of the Glue Grant database. *J Trauma Acute Care Surg*. 2013;74(5):1215–1221;(discussion):1221–1222.

55. Clifton GL, Miller ER, Choi SC, et al. Fluid thresholds and outcome from severe brain injury. *Crit Care Med*. 2002;30(4):739–745.

56. Haut ER, Kalish BT, Cotton BA, et al. Prehospital intravenous fluid administration is associated with higher mortality in trauma patients: a National Trauma Data Bank analysis. *Ann Surg*. 2011;253(2):371–377.

57. Ferrada P, Evans D, Wolfe L, et al. Findings of a randomized controlled trial using limited transthoracic echocardiogram (LTTE) as a hemodynamic monitoring tool in the trauma bay. *J Trauma Acute Care Surg*. 2014;76(1):31–37;(discussion):37–38.

58. Gantner D, Moore EM, Cooper DJ. Intravenous fluids in traumatic brain injury: what's the solution? *Curr Opin Crit Care*. 2014;20(4):385–389.

59. Mangat HS, Chiu YL, Gerber LM, et al. Hypertonic saline reduces cumulative and daily intracranial pressure burdens after severe traumatic brain injury. *J Neurosurg*. 2015;122(1): 202–210.

60 infer S, Bellomo R, Boyce N, et al. A comparison of albumin and saline for fluid resuscitation in the intensive care unit. *N Engl J Med*. 2004;350(22):2247–2256.

61. Mayer J, Boldt J, Poland R, et al. Continuous arterial pressure waveform-based cardiac output using the FloTrac/Vigileo: a review and meta-analysis. *J Cardiothorac Vasc Anesth*. 2009;23(3):401–406.

62. Ferrada P, Murthi S, Anand RJ, et al. Transthoracic focused rapid echocardiographic examination: real-time evaluation of fluid status in critically ill trauma patients. *J Trauma*. 2011;70(1):56–62;(discussion 62–64).

63. Brady HR, Singer GG. Acute renal failure. *Lancet*. 1995;346(8989):1533–1540.

64. Zacharia BE, Ducruet AF, Hickman ZL, et al. Renal dysfunction as an independent predictor of outcome after aneurysmal subarachnoid hemorrhage: a single-center cohort study. *Stroke*. 2009;40(7):2375–2381.

65. Tsagalis G, Akrivos T, Alevizaki M, et al. Long-term prognosis of acute kidney injury after first acute stroke. *Clin J Am Soc Nephrol*. 2009;4(3):616–622.

66. Moore EM, Bellomo R, Nichol A, et al. The incidence of acute kidney injury in patients with traumatic brain injury. *Ren Fail*. 2010;32(9):1060–1065.

67. Davenport A, Will EJ, Davison AM. Early changes in intracranial pressure during haemofiltration treatment in patients with grade 4 hepatic encephalopathy and acute oliguric renal failure. *Nephrol Dial Transplant*. 1990;5(3):192–198.

68. Lin CM, Lin JW, Tsai JT, et al. Intracranial pressure fluctuation during hemodialysis in renal failure patients with intracranial hemorrhage. *Acta Neurochir Suppl*. 2008;101:141–144.

69. Davenport A. Changing the hemodialysis prescription for hemodialysis patients with subdural and intracranial hemorrhage. *Hemodial Int*. 2013;(suppl):S22–27.

70. Davenport A. Renal replacement therapy for the patient with acute traumatic brain injury and severe acute kidney injury. *Contrib Nephrol*. 2007;156:333–339.

71. Fletcher JJ, Bergman K, Carlson G, et al. Continuous renal replacement therapy for refractory intracranial hypertension? *J Trauma*. 2010;68(6):1506–1509.

72. Fletcher JJ, Bergman K, Feucht EC, et al. Continuous renal replacement therapy for refractory intracranial hypertension. *Neurocrit Care*. 2009;11(1):101–105.

73. McCunn M, Reynolds HN, Reuter J, et al. Continuous renal replacement therapy in patients following traumatic injury. *Int J Artif Organs*. 2006;29(2):166–186.

The Role of Intracranial Pressure in Multimodality Monitoring Strategies

9

H. Alex Choi
Suhas S. Bajgur
Tiffany R. Chang

INTRODUCTION

Since intracranial pressure (ICP) and cerebral pressure dynamics were introduced in the 1950s, we have been attempting to simplify their use in the clinical setting. The placement of a fluid-filled catheter into the brain and transducing it with a manometer to measure the pressure inside the cranial vault has led to decades of research into the physiology of the acutely injured brain. Advancements in technology have made numerous devices available to monitor different aspects of cerebral physiology. We now have the ability to measure cerebral pressure variables, blood flow, oxygenation, metabolism, and electrical activity. We are just beginning to understand the complex cerebral physiology of the acutely injured brain.

Although ICP is now routinely monitored as a standard of care in most neurointensive care units, it is unclear if these efforts translate into improved clinical outcomes. The initial studies examining ICP monitoring focused on clinical feasibility and demonstrating an association between high ICP and worse outcome (1). With a number of retrospective and prospective observational studies showing 20 mmHg as a threshold value, guidelines were made, and 20 to 25 mmHg became the cut-off value used in common clinical practice (2,3).

Lost in much of these discussions is the essence of what ICP is really monitoring and how it relates to the information that we are interested in to help our patients. The development of other neuromonitoring techniques has led to questions about combining their measurements with ICP monitoring to individualize treatments. We hope that monitoring additional elements of cerebral physiology and integrating this information with ICP will help in interpreting ICP values and guide therapy to improve patient outcomes.

Why do we measure intracranial pressure?

The first neuromonitoring devices were ICP monitors mainly because of the ease of measurement and the potential therapeutic value. The measurement of ICP is helpful because it correlates with the clinical state the majority of the time. In other words, sicker patients with CT imaging suggesting worse cerebral injury and worse neurological examinations have higher ICPs. The association between higher ICP and clinical outcome is highly reproducible. This has led to widespread clinical use. However, as evidenced by the results of a recent trial, an ICP-guided treatment algorithm has not clearly been associated with improved clinical outcome when compared with a treatment algorithm based on the neurologic examination and radiographic findings (4).

How are the results of the intracranial pressure trial relevant for intracranial pressure monitoring and multimodality monitoring?

Although the ICP trial results are debated, at the very least they demand that we reconsider some of the fundamentals of neuromonitoring. First, monitoring, whether ICP or another modality, has no direct impact on patient outcomes. Therapeutic interventions performed in reaction to neuromonitoring are the only actions that may make a difference in clinical outcomes. The ICP trial is really about the amounts of mannitol, hypertonic saline, vasopressors, sedation, barbiturates, etc. that patients receive. In other words, it is not necessarily the monitor but rather how we respond to the monitor. Second, we need to understand that ICP is only a surrogate marker of what we really want to measure. ICP alone may not be robust enough to represent cerebral physiology and allow us to make clinical decisions that will affect outcomes. In fact, we can ask the question: Why monitor pressure at all? We should take a step back and think about the ideal measurement strategies for the clinician at the bedside. Then we can put ICP in the context of other multimodality monitoring strategies.

What do we want to monitor in patients with acute brain injury?

1. *Cerebral blood volume (CBV):* The need to measure pressure is driven by the need to measure a closely related variable—volume, as the Monro-Kellie doctrine describes. In fact, most of the interpretations of pressure variables are related to volume, such as space-occupying lesions, hemorrhages, edema, and contusions. Most treatments we give patients are also volume related, whether increasing internal jugular venous volume drainage by elevating the head, decreasing CSF volume with an external ventricular drain (EVD), or decreasing cerebral volume using osmotic therapy. Radiographic modalities (CT and MRI) have been the standard method of examining volume. When we look at CT scans, we are looking for space-occupying lesions, such as hemorrhage or edema, that are compressing brain tissue. This suggests that a continuous measurement of cerebral volume would be an important and perhaps even more valuable physiologic monitor than pressure. Changes in ICP should be interpreted with cerebral volume in mind.
2. *Cerebral blood flow (CBF):* Technological advances have allowed us to measure surrogates to CBF and actual CBF, which is perhaps the most important variable to monitor. Using ultrasound technology, transcranial Doppler (TCD) has been used as a surrogate marker of CBF. Devices to measure direct CBF, such as a thermal diffusion probe (TDP), which is inserted into the brain parenchyma, are being developed.
3. *Cerebral oxygenation:* The measurement of cerebral oxygen levels is another advancement that came into use almost as early as pressure monitoring. Studies have shown that invasive cerebral oximetry may be an important determinant of outcome. The invasive nature of the brain tissue oximetry probe severely limits its use, making room for noninvasive cerebral oximetry with near-infrared spectroscopy (NIRS).
4. *Brain activity:* Electroencephalography (EEG) has been traditionally used to detect seizures. More recently, we have begun to think of EEG as a way of monitoring patients for other brain dysfunction, including encephalopathy, ICU delirium, and even ischemia. The advent of intracranial EEG monitoring has brought about the possibility that we have been missing critical information because of the limitations of electrical activity passing through the scalp. Subdural electrocorticography (ECoG) has brought about new ways of monitoring, which have brought to light new pathophysiologic mechanisms for brain injury.

5. *Brain metabolism:* Brain metabolism is closely associated with all of the previous processes. Normal and preserved brain metabolism signifies a healthy state. Altered brain metabolism potentially signifies ongoing cell death. Cerebral microdialysis (MD) has been developed to measure cerebral metabolism continuously. Brain metabolism can also be measured by the amount of oxygen consumed in the brain. Measurements of the saturation of jugular blood as it exits the brain (SjO_2) with a jugular venous catheter are indications of brain metabolism.

All of these markers of cerebral physiology are important to obtain a more complete understanding of the "health" of the acutely injured brain. They are all slightly different in the information that they provide but ultimately are all intertwined.

How does multimodality monitoring change the "one-size-fits-all" approach to intracranial pressure?

Anecdotally, we know that an ICP of 40 mmHg in one patient does not have the same clinical meaning as an ICP of 40 mmHg in another patient. How are we supposed to know if the ICP is dangerous or not? When viewed in the setting of what we would ideally like to measure in our patients with brain injury, ICP is only a part of the equation—and perhaps not even the most important part. In this chapter, we will review the basics of different neuromonitoring techniques and the corollaries of outcomes. We will discuss the clinical translation of current research and point out the strengths and limitations of each technique. Last, we will attempt to describe how using a multimodal monitoring technique can change the one-size-fits-all approach to the management of cerebral physiology to improve clinical outcomes.

MULTIMODALITY MONITORING

Brain Pressure/Volume Measurements

Elevated ICP, especially when refractory to therapy, is associated with a worse clinical outcome (5). However, our basic understanding of the physiology of ICP, the absolute treatment threshold, and the clinical effectiveness of ICP management are still uncertain. Perhaps instead of a generalized threshold for which ICP should be treated, we should be using ICP information to understand cerebral physiology and tailor individualized treatments.

Neuromonitors to measure the brain's ability to regulate CBF and thus brain volume/pressure are one method of individualizing treatment. Cerebral autoregulation is the ability of the brain to regulate the amount of CBF across different blood pressures, or the mean arterial blood pressure (MAP). When cerebral autoregulation is intact, changes in MAP will not affect the volume/pressure in the brain. In this state, no correlation exists between ICP and MAP. When autoregulation is impaired, there is a direct correlation between MAP and volume/pressure. This occurs in both ends of autoregulation, as seen in Figure 9.1. This concept has been functionalized through the development of the pressure autoregulatory index (PRx) (6). The PRx is a correlation between MAP and ICP. When the two are correlated, this means an increase in one is associated with an increase in the other. High PRx correlations are associated with worse outcomes after traumatic brain injury (TBI), intracerebral hemorrhage (ICH), and subarachnoid hemorrhage (SAH) (6–9). By plotting PRx values across different cerebral perfusion pressures (CPPs), a CPP optimum (CPP_{opt}) can be calculated. The CPP_{opt} is the CPP range at which the PRx values are the lowest, usually at the bottom of a U-shaped curve. The magnitude of difference between the actual CPP and the CPP_{opt} in individuals is associated with worse outcomes (9). Identifying CPP_{opt} for an individualized CPP goal and targeting CPP_{opt} may be beneficial for patients. The best method would be to have individualized CPP goals to optimize cerebral autoregulation rather than the population-based goal of CPP measuring 50 to 70 mmHg.

The major limitation to implementation has been the lack of a neuromonitoring infrastructure. The calculation of PRx requires physiologic data at the level of waveform analysis; however, more recent advances may make the PRx concept more available. L-PRx, a similar method using minute-by-minute information and the possibility of measuring ICP continuously through an open EVD, may help with clinical implementation (10,11).

The Monro-Kellie doctrine states that as the volume in the cranial vault increases once beyond the inflection point the pressure increases (Figure 9.2).

We use this concept to measure ICP as a surrogate marker for the measurement of brain volume. The measurement of brain volume is possible with radiographic tests, mostly CT and MRI. However, radiographic tests cannot be performed continuously, which limits their use for bedside monitoring. A continuous monitor for measuring brain volume would be very informative and perhaps clinically useful. A recent study has shown that it is possible to measure brain water content continuously at the bedside. Brain water content is

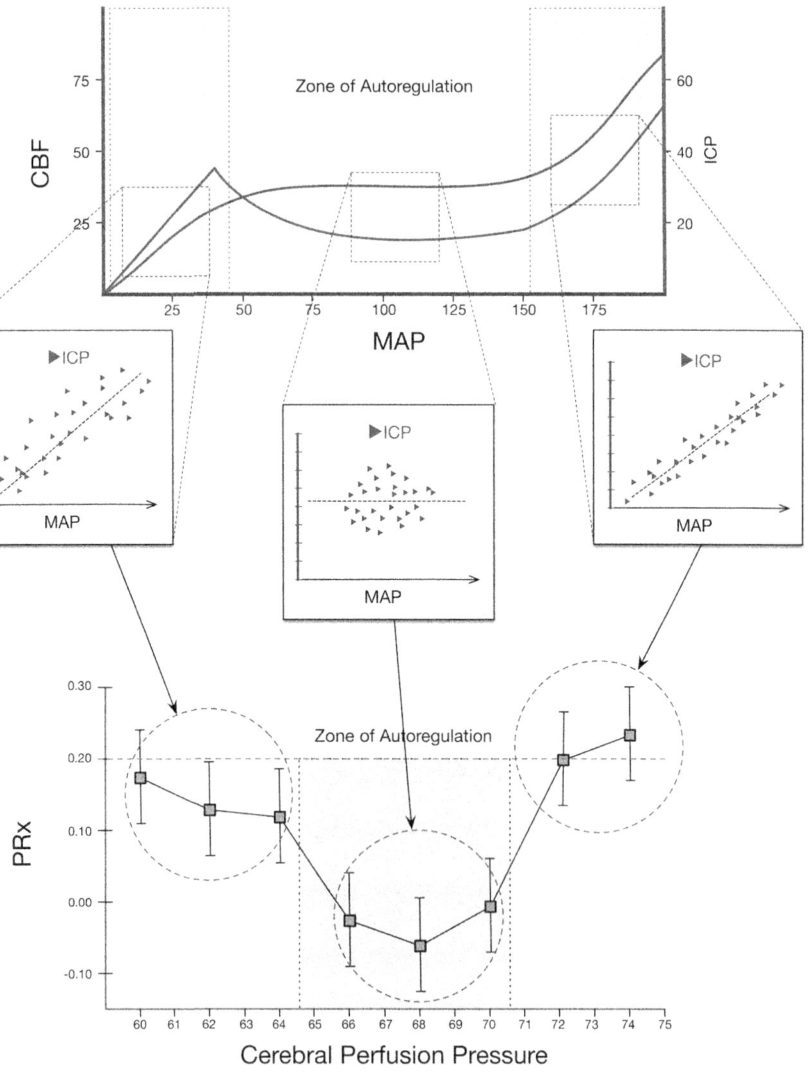

FIGURE 9.1 Intracranial pressure (ICP), mean arterial pressure (MAP), and PRx. *Note:* CBF, cerebral blood flow.

a surrogate marker for brain edema and brain volume. With the use of an intraparenchymal probe that measures the thermal conductivity of the surrounding brain tissue, one can estimate the percentage of water content of the brain tissue (12). This measure of brain edema may be a clinically useful neuromonitoring tool.

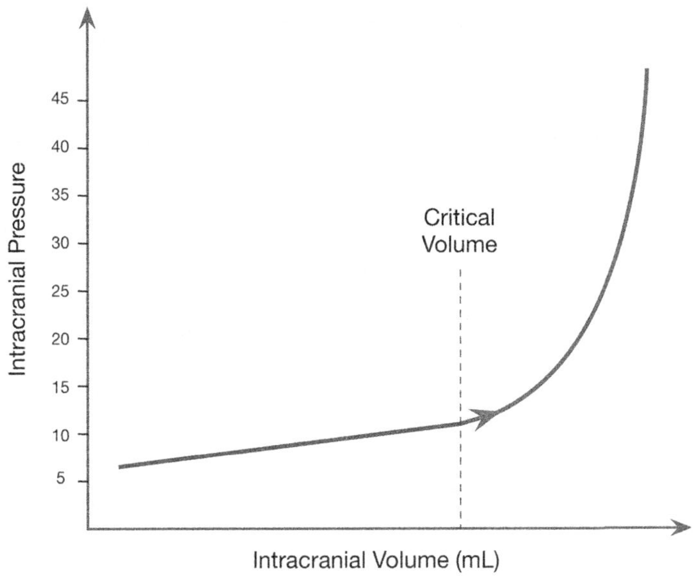

FIGURE 9.2 The Monro-Kellie doctrine.

Cerebral Blood Flow

Cerebral ischemia may be the most important cause of secondary brain injury, making CBF the focus of treatment. Imaging CBF using CT, MR, and PET technologies has made significant advancements. However, technology for the continuous monitoring of real-time CBF is still relatively undeveloped. Most measurements are surrogate measurements of blood flow, with only one technique attempting to measure CBF directly. Cerebral oxygenation and brain oximetry are also surrogate markers of CBF and are most commonly used in clinical practice.

TCD is a noninvasive method of measuring cerebral blood velocity as it passes through large-diameter cerebral blood vessels. The TCD probe emits a high-frequency acoustic signal that penetrates the skull and is reflected back to the probe by flowing blood. The reflected signal gives information about the velocity of the flow. TCD has been studied extensively for use in detecting vasospasm after SAH, showing reasonable sensitivity and specificity for predicting angiographic vasospasm. Threshold values of 120 to 200 cm/min have been used, with the higher thresholds showing better positive predictive values and the lower thresholds useful for negative predictive values (13–15). However, because of the inconsistency of angiographic vasospasm to predict delayed cerebral ischemia (DCI), the ability of TCD to detect DCI is also limited (16).

By integrating TCD with blood pressure waveform information, we have the ability to broaden the utility of TCD. Similar to the PRx, the Mx has been created as an estimation of cerebral autoregulation. It is a moving correlation coefficient between the mean flow velocity of the middle cerebral artery (MCA) and MAP. A high value of this correlation coefficient indicates a loss of cerebral autoregulation (17,18). Critical closing pressure is a concept that uses TCD to measure cerebral vascular resistance. It estimates the theoretical lowest value of arterial blood pressure that is adequate for maintaining CBF. Changes in critical closing pressure during vasospasm and TBI have been reported, but the clinical utility of this estimation of cerebral vascular resistance is unclear (19–21).

The main advantage of TCD is that it is noninvasive, with few side effects. However, it has several significant limitations in that (a) flow velocities measured with TCD are not highly correlated with CBF. For instance, high flow velocities can represent a small constricted blood vessel with decreased CBF (ie, vasospasm) or can represent an increase in blood flow through the same diameter vessel (ie, hyperemia). Using the Lindegaard ratio, which compares the MCA velocities with the ipsilateral carotid velocities, can adjust for these factors. However, this method is also not without problems; (b) another significant confounding factor is that we are only able to measure flow velocities in large cerebral blood vessels, namely the internal carotid arteries, middle cerebral arteries, anterior cerebral arteries, vertebral arteries, and basilar artery. This severely limits information about the dynamics of the distal vasculature. Although attempts have been made to calculate the indices between the systolic and diastolic pressures of the flow velocities to better understand flow dynamics, indices such as the pulsatility index have not been shown to be consistently useful (22); (c) the intermittent nature of the test and the difficulty integrating this information with other physiologic data limits the use of TCD as a bedside monitoring device; and (d) the technique is very operator dependent. The advancement of transcranial color-coded duplex sonography techniques may decrease the interoperator variation and the technical differences, improving accuracy (23). Despite the limitations, TCD is a useful noninvasive test to examine for large-vessel flow dynamics, monitor for microemboli, and screen for significant proximal vessel vasospasm after SAH (24).

A more direct measure of CBF is possible with the use of a TDP, Hemedex®. Inserting a probe into the brain to measure thermal diffusion and the power needed to keep the temperature of the probe constant can calculate thermal diffusion cerebral blood flow (TDCBF). Intraoperative studies examining TDCBF have shown it to accurately reflect absolute CBF (25,26). TDCBF values have also been shown to decrease before and during significant vasospasm (27).

Cerebral autoregulation can be measured more directly with a CBF monitor. A scatter plot of CBF and CPP can reproduce the autoregulation curve. CPP goals can then be directed at goal CBF values. The flow-related autoregulation index (FRx), mirroring the PRx, is a moving correlation between CBF and CPP (28). Studies using FRx to predict neurologic outcomes are too preliminary at this point for use in the routine clinical setting (29).

The advantage of the Hemedex® is that it measures CBF in units of milliliters per 100 grams of brain tissue. Additionally, the possibility of using the same probe to calculate CBF and brain water content is attractive (12). However, the disadvantages have limited its wide use in clinical practice. Mainly, the regional measurement of CBF emphasizes the importance of location placement of the probe. The stability of the probe and the frequent recalibrations are also issues. More research examining actual TDCBF thresholds are required for wider adoption of this technology in routine clinical practice.

Cerebral Oxygenation

The most widely used invasive oximetry tool is the measurement of the partial pressure of brain tissue oxygen tension using the Licox® catheter. Normal values for brain tissue oxygen have been identified as approximately equal to 30 mmHg (30). Similar to our approach with ICP, studies have shown that lower $PbtO_2$ values are associated with worse clinical outcomes. Proposed thresholds have been 8, 10, 15, and 20 mmHg. The most agreed-upon threshold for which treatment is necessary is 20 mmHg (31–33). $PbtO_2$ represents a balance between oxygen delivery (a function of PaO_2 and CBF), oxygen consumption, and oxygen diffusion. The determinants of $PbtO_2$ have been well studied. Factors that influence $PbtO_2$ include the partial pressure of dissolved oxygen in the blood around the probe (PaO_2), CBF, the hemoglobin-carrying capacity, the diffusion of oxygen, and brain metabolism (34,35).

The management of $PbtO_2$ has two overlapping but slightly separate strategies. It is generally used as a monitor for cerebral oxygenation, with the focus on providing adequate oxygen tension to brain tissue. $PbtO_2$ information can also be used as a surrogate marker for CBF. A falling $PbtO_2$ can signify a number of processes, such as an expanding hematoma causing worsening perihematomal edema, vasospasm after SAH causing worsening ischemia, or continued

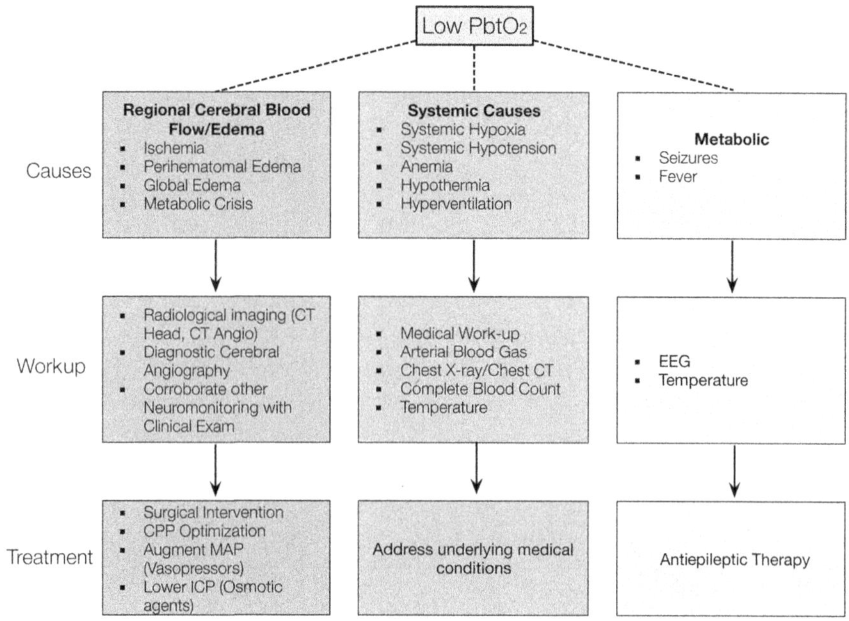

FIGURE 9.3 Approach to management of low $PbtO_2$. *Note:* CPP, central perfusion pressure; EEG, electroencephalogram; ICP, intracranial pressure.

ongoing seizures. When faced with a dropping $PbtO_2$, the most important action is to determine the cause and tailor the treatment to it (Figure 9.3).

Broadly, there are three reasons for decreasing $PbtO_2$ values. First, a decrease in the regional CBF or an increase in cerebral edema can cause issues with the diffusion of oxygen. Elevated ICP and cerebral edema will both cause a local decrease in CBF and cause a decrease in $PbtO_2$. The workup consists of identifying the potential causes for neurologic deterioration, similar to the workup for a patient with a worsening neurologic examination. Cerebral ischemia from vascular lesions or from cerebral edema should be investigated. Especially in the setting of SAH treatment, a decreasing $PbtO_2$ may suggest clinically significant vasospasm. Second, systemic causes for a low $PbtO_2$ should be addressed. As PaO_2 is the main driver of $PbtO_2$, and hyperventilation is a main driver of low $PbtO_2$, an arterial blood gas (ABG) and other medical workups should be performed. Third, increases in brain metabolism can decrease $PbtO_2$ values. Seizures are associated with a low $PbtO_2$; however, the changes are small and may be difficult to detect (36).

Is increasing the FIO_2 to increase $PbtO_2$ a good clinical strategy?

Although low $PbtO_2$ has been associated with a worse outcome, it is still not clear if a $PbtO_2$-guided treatment strategy will improve outcomes. The PaO_2 is clearly the strongest determinant of $PbtO_2$, meaning that increasing FIO_2 will increase the $PbtO_2$ dramatically. This is in fact one way to test proper functioning of the $PbtO_2$ monitor; by increasing the FIO_2 to 100% briefly, you will get a dramatic rise in the $PbtO_2$.

Whether increasing FIO_2 has positive effects on brain metabolism is controversial. In general, there is conflicting evidence about whether normobaric hyperoxia is beneficial for brain tissue and clinical outcomes. Although previous studies have suggested a benefit from hyperoxia, more recent studies have shown that hyperoxia may be bad for the brain. Studies of patients with ischemic stroke, SAH, TBI, and cardiac arrest have all shown that hyperoxia is associated with worse neurologic outcomes (37–39). None of these studies included $PbtO_2$ monitoring, but we can conjecture that if they had, patients with hyperoxia would have had higher numbers and possibly fewer brain hypoxemia events. One thing to keep in mind is that hyperoxia causes a decrease in regional CBF by causing vasoconstriction; this occurs as a result of decreased carbon dioxide secondary to superoxygenated hemoglobin, ie, the Haldane effect.

Additionally, multimodality studies have questioned the effect of hyperoxia on brain metabolism. Some have reported that hyperoxia does not affect or possibly worsens brain metabolism, while others cite a benefit (40,41). Overall, the summary of studies suggests that increases in PaO_2 will increase $PbtO_2$ levels, but this does not necessarily translate into an improved metabolic state (42,43). Studies looking at hyperbaric oxygen for the treatment of TBI are ongoing but are too preliminary and costly to have an impact on routine clinical practice at this time (44). Given the controversy, some will use an increase in FIO_2 as a last resort to treat low $PbtO_2$ values.

Does $PbtO_2$-guided treatment improve outcomes?

Although multiple studies have shown improved outcomes with the use of $PbtO_2$ monitoring, they all have significant flaws. No definitive statements can be made about the effect of $PbtO_2$ monitoring on clinical outcomes. The Benefits of Oxygen Saturation Targeting (BOOST) II trial is an ongoing randomized clinical trial that hypothesizes that a treatment protocol using

Licox® monitoring will decrease the amount of time that $PbtO_2$ values are below the critical threshold of 20 mmHg. This is one of the first large-scale studies to attempt to test neuromonitoring for its effects on clinical outcome. Likely, the results will show that we are able to keep $PbtO_2$ values above the threshold more often when monitored, as they are easily observed at the bedside. By targeting higher CPPs and higher PaO_2 levels, $PbtO_2$ values are expected to respond. However, whether this will translate to improved clinical outcomes is the real question. Findings about the secondary clinical outcomes will be important indicators of the impact of $PbtO_2$ monitoring.

How does brain tissue oximetry relate to intracranial pressure?

The relationship between $PbtO_2$ and ICP is not linear, as they measure separate phenomena. The relationship varies on many factors but mainly on the state of autoregulation. Assuming that PaO_2, PCO_2, and hemoglobin (Hb) are stable, if autoregulation in the region of interest is intact then no significant relationship exists between $PbtO_2$ and CPP; ie, when CPP is increased or decreased the brain should autoregulate flow and maintain $PbtO_2$ levels. If there is loss of autoregulation, as CPP increases so does $PbtO_2$. This relationship works inversely with ICP. If autoregulation is lost, an increase in ICP leads to a decrease in CPP and a decrease in $PbtO_2$. This relationship can be used to our advantage for identifying cerebral autoregulation using $PbtO_2$ values and CPP values. A simple scatter plot can approximate cerebral autoregulation by looking at $PbtO_2$ values across CPP (Figure 9.4).

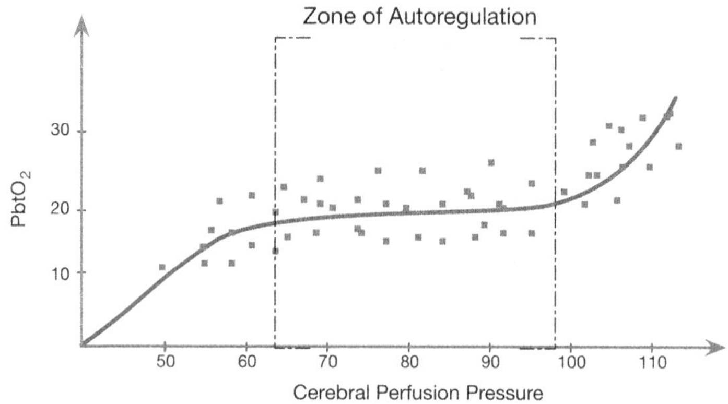

FIGURE 9.4 Relationship between $PbtO_2$ and central perfusion pressure (CPP).

How does hypothermia change $PbtO_2$?

Hypothermia decreases $PbtO_2$ values. Some have hypothesized that decreased ICP associated with hypothermia would lead to higher $PbtO_2$ values. However, one must remember that hypothermia decreases ICP by decreasing cerebral metabolic demand and decreasing CBF. Decreased CBF leads to a decrease in $PbtO_2$. When examining a subset of the National Acute Brain Injury Study: Hypothermia (NABISH) I and NABISH II trial subjects, those who were treated with therapeutic hypothermia had lower $PbtO_2$ values than subjects who were treated with normothermia (Figure 9.5) (45).

This phenomenon can be seen at the bedside. When rapidly cooling a patient, the $PbtO_2$ tends to decrease. However, this does not mean that therapeutic hypothermia is bad for the brain. When hypothermic, the brain's metabolism is decreased, which is the premise for the neuroprotective effects of hypothermia. Likely, therapeutic hypothermia is associated with a decreased need for oxygen as well. It is plausible that the threshold for cerebral hypoxia in the hypothermic brain is different than the normothermic brain, and the hypothermic brain may be able to tolerate lower $PbtO_2$ values.

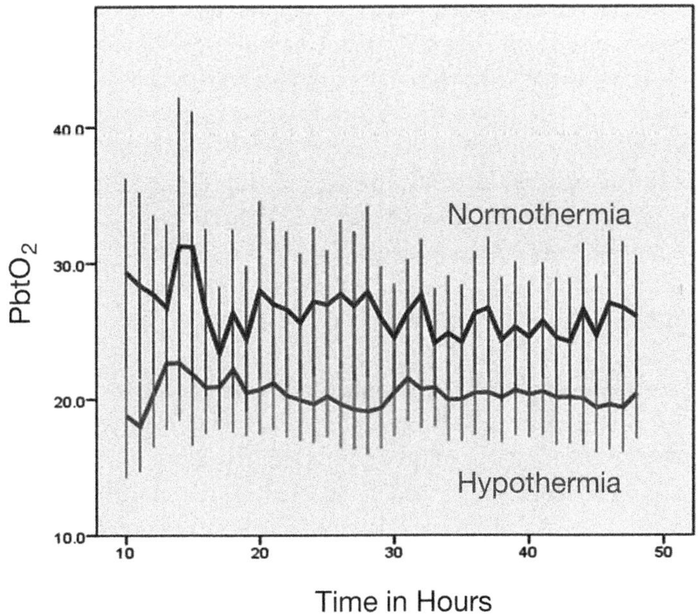

FIGURE 9.5 Difference between $PbtO_2$ in normothermic and hypothermic patients after traumatic brain injury (TBI). *Note:* Presented at the Neurocritical Care Society meeting 2013.

There are several common pitfalls to avoid:

1. *Treating decreasing $PbtO_2$ values without understanding the cause and addressing it appropriately.* As $PbtO_2$ decreases, the simple action of increasing the FIO_2 may resolve the situation, and no further investigation is performed. This is not the correct method of dealing with a falling $PbtO_2$ value. The etiology of a $PbtO_2$ drop needs to be adequately investigated and addressed simultaneously with actions to increase the $PbtO_2$ value.
2. *Threshold management is another potential pitfall.* Like ICP monitoring, patients with lower $PbtO_2$ values generally have worse outcomes, but this is not universally true. Individuals likely have different thresholds that lead to further brain injury. A change of $PbtO_2$ from 35 mmHg to 20 mmHg may be as significant as a change from 25 to 15. However, if we are focused on 20 mmHg as a threshold we will not respond to this vital information appropriately.
3. *The side effect of optimal $PbtO_2$ management can cause significant medical complications.* Methods of increasing $PbtO_2$, such as inducing hypertension to increase CPP to greater than 70 mmHg, administering hypertonic saline to decrease ICP, and giving blood transfusions to maintain higher Hb levels, all increase the risk of pulmonary complications (46). I have witnessed patients in florid pulmonary edema receiving vasopressors for higher MAPs and blood transfusions to increase Hb in response to low $PbtO_2$ values. This is probably not appropriate care. When focusing on neuromonitoring values without being attentive to the general medical condition of patients, it is easy to lose sight of the basic principles of critical care.
4. *Hypothermia is a cause of low $PbtO_2$.* Hypothermia causes a decrease in metabolism, which is coupled with a decrease in CBF. This will cause a decrease in $PbtO_2$. It is unclear whether a decreased $PbtO_2$ value in the setting of hypothermia is harmful.

NIRS is a noninvasive and easily applied method of neuromonitoring. NIRS technology uses the differences in absorption coefficients of oxyhemoglobin and deoxyhemoglobin to monitor oxygen saturation. A sticker is placed on the forehead, and a probe emits light that is reflected by the brain, which another probe detects. There has been considerable concern that contamination of the signal from superficial tissues causes inaccurate values. Additionally, clear thresholds for care have not been well established. Current research has focused on using NIRS as a trend monitor to examine cerebral autoregulatory status. A recent study used NIRS to measure disturbances in autoregulation by correlating NIRS values with changes in MAP (47). However, this type of analysis requires an integrated monitoring system that is not readily available. The routine clinical use of NIRS to detect secondary brain injury and guide treatment decisions is probably premature at this point.

Brain Metabolism

The Brain Trauma Foundation and the Neurocritical Care Society endorse the monitoring of jugular venous saturation (SjO_2) (2). SjO_2 is a measurement of the oxygenation of the blood that is exiting the brain. This information reflects the oxygenation entering the brain (primarily the PaO_2 and the amount of CBF) and the brain's use of oxygen (the brain metabolism of oxygen). Values lower than 55% and higher than 75% have been associated with poor outcomes. Low values suggest that the brain is being hypoperfused or is hypermetabolic. High values indicate decreased brain metabolism resulting in shunting of oxygen through extensively damaged brain tissue. By measuring SjO_2 and the arterial PaO_2, we can quantify the difference between oxygen delivery and oxygen uptake, which is a surrogate measure of brain metabolism. However, studies have been inconclusive about the efficacy of using SjO_2 and its impact on outcomes. In addition, the lack of the development of dedicated catheters for monitoring jugular venous saturation causes relatively higher failure rates for jugular catheters than for other monitors.

Low SjO_2 values should be approached similarly to low $PbtO_2$ reads. The systemic reasons for a low SjO_2, which include hypoxia and increased systemic metabolism, should be investigated. Simultaneously, the reasons for brain hypoperfusion and increased brain metabolism should be investigated and addressed. Interventions to increase CBF, including CPP optimization, should be performed.

Microdialysis (MD) has been used for decades to monitor chemistries in different organs in vivo. Cerebral MD is used to measure the concentration of small molecules in the brain parenchyma. A very thin catheter with a semipermeable membrane (20 kDa or 100 kDa) is placed in the interstitial tissue of the brain. A dialysate fluid is slowly pumped through the catheter and comes into equilibrium with the extracellular fluid. A small tube collects the dialysate fluid that can be analyzed; this is usually done every hour but can be collected as often as every 20 minutes. The idea is to get a measure of the metabolic status of the brain tissue. The most well-studied markers are pyruvate, lactate, and glucose. Other molecules are now being measured, including glutamate, glycerol, inflammatory cytokines, amino acids, and electrolytes, but the interpretations of these values are not well established. Glucose is the major fuel source for the brain. Glucose is metabolized to pyruvate and in the presence of oxygen enters the Kreb's cycle to produce adenosine triphosphate

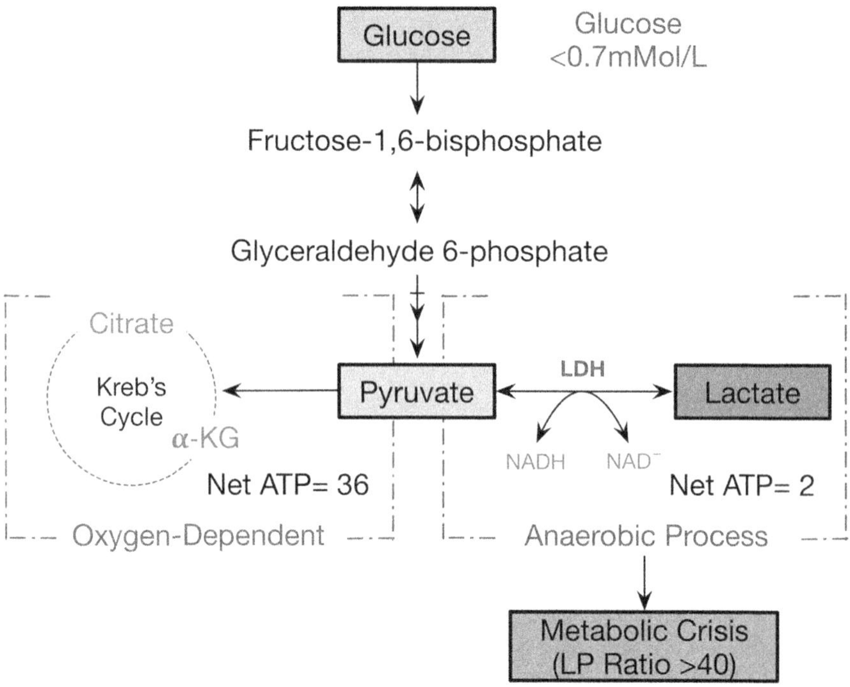

FIGURE 9.6 Biochemical basis of cerebral microdialysis.

(ATP). In the absence of oxygen, pyruvate is transformed to lactate. The balance between lactate and pyruvate indicates whether the cells are undergoing aerobic or anaerobic respiration. This version of biochemistry is clearly oversimplified. The interpretation of metabolism that MD measures is complex (Figure 9.6).

High levels of lactate, low levels of pyruvate, and low levels of glucose are generally associated with worse clinical outcomes. A term called *metabolic crisis* (MC) has been coined to represent a poor metabolic state of the brain. MC is associated with high lactate and low pyruvate, specifically with a lactate to pyruvate ratio (LPR) greater than 40 and brain glucose less than 0.7 mmol/L. High lactate (representing anaerobic respiration) and low pyruvate and glucose (representing low fuel for the brain) suggest that metabolism is increased in the setting of low oxygen and glucose delivery. The extent to which MD is clinically helpful at the bedside is unclear. Mainly, this is because the determinants of MD values are not well understood. Likely, microdialysate chemicals represent a balance between metabolism and energy. Due to the complexity of ascertaining the exact cause of changes in microdialysate values, it is difficult to know which physiologic parameters to treat. For example, when the LPR is high it is often unclear as to what intervention is necessary to improve it.

How should I approach a worsening lactate to pyruvate ratio?

In general, a rising LPR is analogous to a worsening neurologic examination and should be treated in the same manner, by examining the possible etiologies. These include ischemia, worsening cerebral edema, seizures, and other causes of secondary brain injury (48–52). Interventions focus on decreasing metabolic demand (avoiding fever and treating seizures) and increasing the delivery of necessary fuel (avoiding hyperventilation, optimizing CPP, and avoiding hypoglycemia).

Although an increasing LPR may be associated with a clinical change, its ability (the sensitivity or positive predictive value) to predict clinically relevant events is yet to be confirmed. Often, a workup for an elevated LPR is unrevealing. Complicating the situation is the fact that in some instances an elevated LPR is associated with improving neurologic status. Although LPR has been shown to be a reasonable predictor of clinical outcomes, it is unclear if LPR is a modifiable risk factor (49).

What about worsening brain glucose?

One easily modifiable variable that MD detects is brain glucose levels. Because serum glucose and brain glucose levels are closely correlated, changes in serum glucose are reflected in brain glucose levels. Tight glycemic control has been shown to be associated with more episodes of MC, as lower serum glucose values have been associated with low brain glucose values. As suggested in the past, these findings have been used to support the idea that tight glucose control may be especially harmful to brain tissue in brain-injured patients (51). How this translates to patient outcomes is not clear.

How does metabolic failure relate to intracranial pressure?

There is an association between high LPR, low brain glucose, and higher ICP values (8,50). However, treating ICP or treating MC may or may not resolve the other. Whether the association is causative is truly unclear. As sicker patients tend to have higher ICP and are more frequently in MC, they both may be markers of the severity of disease. Further studies on the treatment of MC and its impact on ICP and vice versa are needed.

Electrical Activity

Classically, EEG and continuous EEG (cEEG) have been used to detect seizures. More recently, EEG has been used for the neuromonitoring of patients with acute brain injury. The increased utilization of cEEG for monitoring patients with acute brain injury and other encephalopathies has shown that even in systemic disease, cEEG can detect abnormal activity that can potentially worsen brain injury (53). Studies of patients with acute brain injury, SAH, or ICH have shown an alarmingly high rate of ictal patterns on EEG. These patterns have been associated with worse outcomes, leading some to call for their aggressive treatment (52,54,55). cEEG has also been used to detect cerebral ischemia after SAH. Changes in the ratio between fast frequencies and slower frequencies (alpha/delta ratio) have been associated with DCI (56). The detection of these patterns and its associated impact on outcome, paired with an increased availability of continuous monitoring, has led to cEEG monitoring in patients who have primarily systemic disease, ie, sepsis. Patients with sepsis and critical illness in surgical and medical ICUs have also shown a significant amount of abnormal ictal patterns and similar associations with poor outcome (53,57,58).

The advantage of cEEG monitoring is its noninvasive, continuous nature. The disadvantage is the need for equipment and manpower to continually place and maintain leads and read the EEG. The automation of cEEG reading with more complex algorithms will help resolve some of these problems.

Intracranial monitoring for electrical activity

A major challenge with scalp EEG monitoring is the need for the brain's electrical activity to pass through bone and soft tissue so that surface electrodes can read it. To detect a seizure on the surface of the scalp, at least 10 to 20 cm^2 of cerebral cortex must fire in synchrony (59). Abnormal electrical activity below this threshold may go completely undetected. Other challenges include electrode contact with skin, muscle artifact, and interference from other electrical devices, leading to poor signal-to-noise ratio, especially in critically ill patients who are surrounded by electrical devices. This phenomenon is often demonstrated in patients who have ongoing clinical complex partial seizures and improve with benzodiazepine treatment and antiepileptic drugs (AEDs) without a clear surface EEG correlate (60).

To test the possibility that abnormal electrical activity may be occurring that a scalp EEG cannot detect, intracranial monitoring has been developed. Intracortical EEG consists of a single electrode placed into the parenchyma of the brain to detect abnormal electrical activity. Early experience with this technique has shown it to be safe and informative. Numerous examples of abnormal ictal patterns have been detected on intracortical monitoring with very few seen on scalp EEG. The presence of ictal patterns on intracortical EEG has been associated with worse LPR seen on MD and worse clinical outcomes. In addition, ictal patterns on intracortical EEG have been associated with changes in heart rate, blood pressure, and respiratory rate, suggesting that these subclinical electrical events exert a physiologic effect (61,36). Several factors limit the widespread use of intracortical EEG. The clinical significance of ictal patterns seen only in intracortical EEG is still controversial. Although these patterns portend worse outcomes, they may simply be corollaries to worse brain injury, and the administration of AEDs may only lead to additional side effects and unnecessary treatments. On the other hand, they may be ictal patterns leading to secondary brain injury, and treatment could improve clinical outcomes. Further studies are required to answer these important questions. In addition, the need for experienced technicians, neurointensivists, and epileptologists to interpret the signals and their potential clinical correlates limits the spread of this technology at this time.

Electrocorticography

Cortical spreading depression (CSD), measured by electrocorticography, was first described in the 1940s and has since been primarily studied in the pathophysiology of migraine headaches. It describes a wave of neuronal depolarization associated with an influx of cations and water. This wave of depolarization spreads cortically and is associated with a wave of hyperemia. Following this wave of activity is a wave of a decrease in cerebral blood. After acute brain injury, CSD has been shown to trigger a state of cortical spreading ischemia and predicts clinical seizures. It is associated with worse outcomes after TBI and SAH (62–66).

Similar to other multimodality techniques, we have little proof that treating CSD will indeed improve clinical outcomes. Medications such as ketamine and others have been proposed to decrease the number of CSDs, but more studies are needed (67). In addition, the need for a craniotomy to place subcortical leads, the expertise needed for the placement, and the complexity of monitoring and interpretation severely limits the utilization of electrocorticography. More recently, however, cortical scalp EEG correlates to CSD have been described, which may allow for more studies and more widespread use (68).

A SUMMARY OF MULTIMODALITY MONITORING

In the absence of a reliable neurologic examination, the ability to monitor the health of an injured brain is severely limited. The goal is to detect and

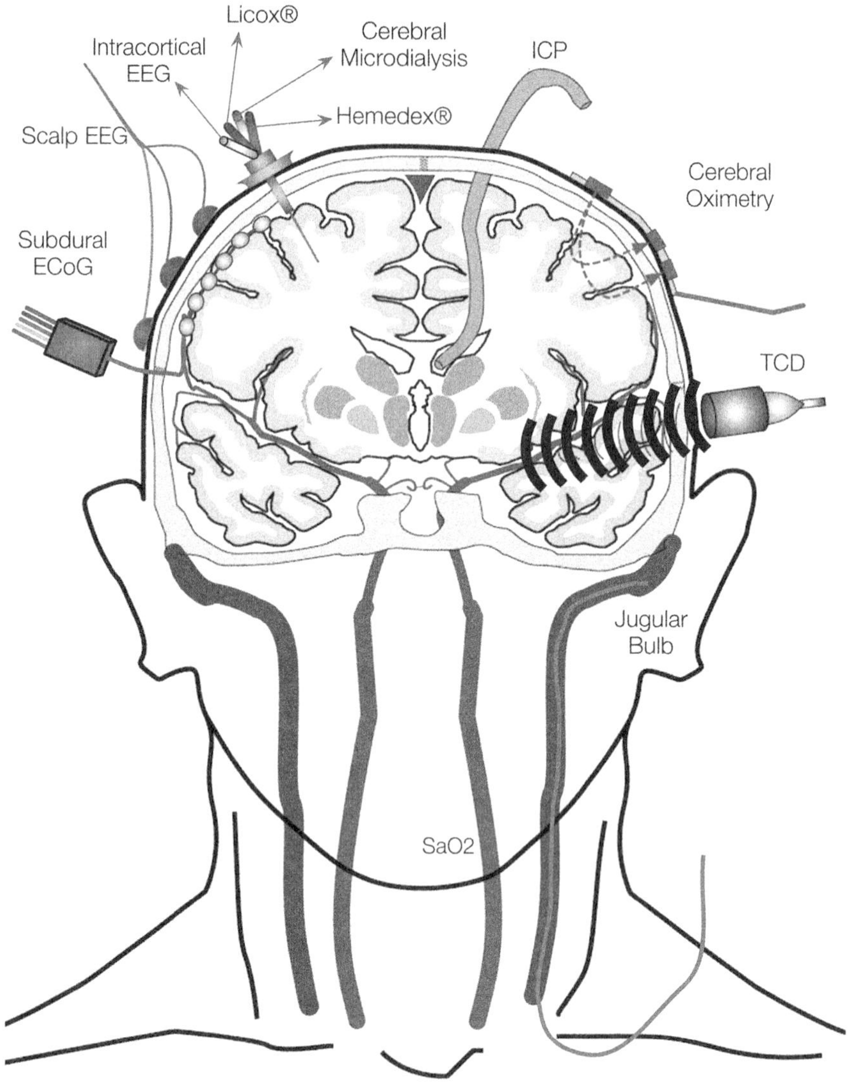

FIGURE 9.7 Multimodality monitoring in the neurocritical care unit. *Note:* EEG, electroencephalogram; ECoG, electrocorticography; ICP, intracranial pressure; TCD, transcranial Doppler.

prevent secondary brain injury. Because multimodality monitoring is used as a surrogate marker in the neurologic examination, a general principle is that changes in neuromonitoring values should be responded to with changes in neurologic examinations. For an overview of monitoring modalities, see Figure 9.7.

The guidelines for neuromonitoring are mostly based on expert opinion and observational studies. Few studies investigating the effect of monitoring on clinical outcomes have been performed, and most are of poor quality. The conclusion from a recent consensus conference emphasized that "ICP management has the potential to influence outcome, particularly when care is targeted and individualized and supplemented with data from other monitors including clinical examination and imaging." It stressed the need for adjustments due to the limited predictive value of ICP and suggested that 20 mmHg is not appropriate for all patients. Multimodality monitoring may help identify acceptable ICP in individual patients (69).

Often, when clinical information about a patient is difficult to interpret, it is natural to try to collect more data in terms of additional history, additional laboratory measurements, or in this case, more physiologic information. As we have reviewed in this chapter, a number of monitoring devices are available for use, each with its own specific monitoring capabilities, advantages, and disadvantages.

Practical Advice for Selecting Patients for Multimodality Monitoring

Which patients should I monitor?

Most would agree that the neurologic examination is the gold standard for monitoring patients. Patients who do not have a consistent, reproducible examination should be considered for invasive neuromonitoring. Most studies using neuromonitoring have been performed in the TBI and the SAH populations. However, any patient who has a severe brain injury and is at risk for secondary injury should be monitored. Increasingly, patients with ICH, cardiac arrest, and acute liver failure are being studied and could be considered for neuromonitoring.

Which invasive devices should I choose?

When selecting patients for multimodality monitoring, the key is to identify the complication that you are trying to detect and treat. The most commonly used modality is $PbtO_2$ monitoring. If you were to choose one modality, $PbtO_2$ is most likely to change the management of the patient due to a) it helps us to understand the determinants of brain oxygenation; b) it is the monitor with the most clear-cut treatment algorithms; and c) in addition to threshold-based treatment strategies, it is capable of cerebral autoregulation studies.

MD monitoring can be very informative and perhaps has the most robust research potential. However, the practical difficulties and costs associated with the machine and the additional nursing care required prohibit its routine use. In addition, the clear determinants of LPR are not understood, and the complexity of the monitoring device leads to difficulties in knowing how to appropriately react to changes in LPR. The only exceptions are brain glucose levels. The ability to control brain glucose levels by adjusting serum glucose levels makes this a potentially very useful tool, but studies need to be performed to validate this practice. The Hemedex® probe has the advantage of measuring CBF, which may be the most important physiologic parameter, and its potential for measuring cerebral brain water content makes this technology very attractive. However, until more research is performed to validate its clinical utility, its use is also limited.

Where should the monitor be placed?

With such monitoring, we must remember that invasive probes monitor the cerebral physiology in a small region of brain tissue. This has led to much speculation regarding the effectiveness of invasive monitoring. All information obtained must be interpreted with this in mind. In patients with a diffuse process, including severe TBI without a focal lesion or a high-grade SAH with a poor exam, invasive monitors should be placed in the nondominant frontal lobe between the anterior cerebral artery (ACA)/MCA territories. In these cases, optimizing the local region of monitoring should translate to a favorable environment for the entire brain. In a disease with local disruption, an attempt should be made to place the probe in tissue most at risk for further damage. For instance, in patients with ICH or TBI with focal lesions, tissue at risk in the perihematoma/pericontusion area should be monitored. This is an important concept because of the regional nature of the information that is gained. For instance, if your right arm was at risk for compartment syndrome because of a fracture but your monitor is placed in the left arm, by the time your monitor detected a problem it would be too late. This concept applies to the brain as well.

A Practical Algorithmic Approach to Intracranial Pressure Management in Patients Undergoing Multimodality Monitoring: When to Tolerate Intracranial Pressure Elevation and When to Treat

Multimodality monitoring has been plagued by research that has used other multimodality agents as end points. Threshold treatments, ie, treating to make sure a value is above or below a certain number, may not be the best method of using multimodality data. Although treatment thresholds of ICP greater than

20 mmHg, $PbtO_2$ less than 20 mmHg, CBF less than 15 to 18 mL/g/sec, LPR greater than 40, and cerebral glucose less than 0.7 mmol/L are used for treatment, this does not represent an individualized approach. The very advantage of multimodality monitoring is the ability to collect a robust amount of information for a specific patient at a specific time. Threshold treatments are based on population information—the idea that most patients are similar and that if we apply the same goals across the board patients will do better. The use of universal threshold-based management strips much of the advantage that we gain by using multimodality monitoring. The alternative is a treatment strategy that uses individualized thresholds for patient-specific goals. Much like the movement for individualized medicine in pharmacology or in cancer treatment, we now have the ability to individualize therapy in the neurocritical care unit.

An example of individualized medicine is the ability to optimize MAP and ICP, depending on other physiologic monitors, to define cerebral autoregulatory curves. By using simple scatter plots (ICP vs. MAP, $PbtO_2$ vs. MAP, and CBF vs. MAP) we can attempt to recreate the cerebral autoregulation curve (Figure 9.8). By using PRx, ORx, and FRx graphs, we will be able to identify the optimum CPP for which autoregulation is most intact.

MD is a more difficult modality to threshold because we are still not completely sure of the determinants of lactate, pyruvate, and other chemicals. The practical way of using MD information is for the early detection of something going wrong. Levels of serum glucose very clearly affect cerebral glucose, however. Some have used cerebral glucose thresholds to adjust serum glucose levels.

FUTURE DIRECTIONS

1. Efforts to integrate information from different monitors and display information in an easy-to-interpret, meaningful way need to occur to make clinical decision making at the bedside easier.
2. We need to move beyond simple threshold management to identifying individualized treatment algorithms.
3. Further work in noninvasive monitoring will make multimodality monitoring safer and feasible for more patients.
4. Research in multimodality monitoring should focus on examining the acute cerebral physiologic effects of bedside interventions to better understand our therapies. The physiology of mannitol, hypertonic saline, nimodipine, and therapeutic hypothermia are all interventions that are commonly used, but their cerebral physiologic effects at the bedside are not well understood.

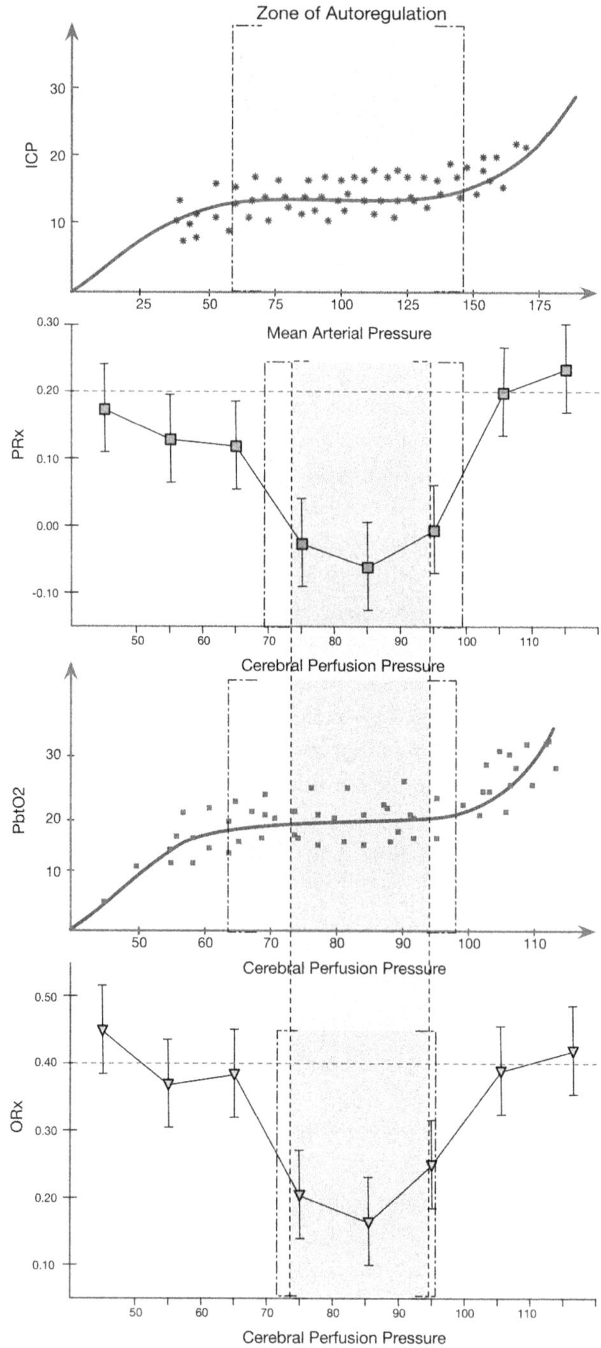

FIGURE 9.8 Composite neuromonitoring of mean arterial pressure (MAP), intracranial pressure (ICP), $PbtO_2$, PRx, and ORx.

5. Multimodality monitoring can be used to better understand the physiology of the acutely injured brain.
6. Multimodality monitoring can help identify and understand new pathophysiologic processes, such as CSD. The identification of new pathophysiologic processes will help to identify new targets of interventions.

CONCLUSIONS

The use of multimodality monitoring enhances our understanding of brain physiology. ICP should be used as one component of a multimodality strategy. The use of information integration and analytics is essential to the advancement of clinical care. A focus on individualized, physiology-based treatment strategies is essential for translating our understanding of the brain to effective clinical treatments.

References

1. Lundberg N, Troupp H, Lorin H. Continuous recording of the ventricular-fluid pressure in patients with severe acute traumatic brain injury. A preliminary report. *J Neurosurg*. 1965;22(6):581–590.

2. Le Roux P, Menon DK, Citerio G, et al. Consensus summary statement of the International Multidisciplinary Consensus Conference on Multimodality Monitoring in Neurocritical Care: a statement for healthcare professionals from the Neurocritical Care Society and the European Society of Intensive Care Medicine. *Intensive Care Med*. 2014;282–296.

3. Brain Trauma Foundation. *Guidelines for the Management of Severe Traumatic Brain Injury 3rd Edition. Neurotrauma*. 2007; 24(suppl 1):S1–S106.

4. Chesnut RM, Temkin N, Carney N, et al. A trial of intracranial-pressure monitoring in traumatic brain injury. *N Engl J Med*. 2012;367(26):2471–2481.

5. Treggiari MM, Schutz N, Yanez ND, et al. Role of intracranial pressure values and patterns in predicting outcome in traumatic brain injury: a systematic review. *Neurocrit Care*. 2007;6(2):104–112.

6. Czosnyka M, Smielewski P, Kirkpatrick P, et al. Continuous assessment of the cerebral vasomotor reactivity in head injury. *Neurosurgery*. 1997;41(1):11–17;(discussion):17–19. 7. Eide PK, Sorteberg A, Bentsen G, et al. Pressure-derived versus pressure wave amplitude–derived indices of cerebrovascular pressure reactivity in relation to early clinical state and 12-month outcome following aneurysmal subarachnoid hemorrhage. *J Neurosurg*. 2012;116(5): 961–971.

8. Ko S-B, Choi HA, Parikh G, et al. Multimodality monitoring for cerebral perfusion pressure optimization in comatose patients with intracerebral hemorrhage. *Stroke*. 2011;42(11): 3087–3092.

9. Steiner LA, Czosnyka M, Piechnik SK, et al. Continuous monitoring of cerebrovascular pressure reactivity allows determination of optimal cerebral perfusion pressure in patients with traumatic brain injury. *Crit Care Med*. 2002;30(4):733–738.

10. Lang EW, Kasprowicz M, Smielewski P, et al. Short pressure reactivity index versus long pressure reactivity index in the management of traumatic brain injury. March 2015; 122:588–594.

11. Aries MJH, de Jong SF, van Dijk JMC, et al. Observation of autoregulation indices during ventricular CSF drainage after aneurysmal subarachnoid hemorrhage: a pilot study. *Neurocrit Care.* 2015;23(3):347–354.

12. Ko S-B, Choi HA, Parikh G, et al. Real time estimation of brain water content in comatose patients. *Ann Neurol.* 2012;72(3):344–350.

13. Suarez JI, Qureshi AI, Yahia AB, et al. Symptomatic vasospasm diagnosis after subarachnoid hemorrhage: evaluation of transcranial Doppler ultrasound and cerebral angiography as related to compromised vascular distribution. *Crit Care Med.* 2002;30(6):1348–1355.

14. Kincaid MS, Souter MJ, Treggiari MM, et al. Accuracy of transcranial Doppler ultrasonography and single-photon emission computed tomography in the diagnosis of angiographically demonstrated cerebral vasospasm. *J Neurosurg.* 2009;110:67–72.

15. Vora YY, Suarez-Almazor M, Steinke DE, Martin ML, Findlay JM. Role of transcranial Doppler monitoring in the diagnosis of cerebral vasospasm after subarachnoid hemorrhage. *Neurosurgery.* 1999;44(6):1237–1238.

16. Carrera E, Schmidt JM, Oddo M, et al. Transcranial Doppler for predicting delayed cerebral ischemia after subarachnoid hemorrhage. *Neurosurgery.* 2009;65(2):314–316.

17. Calviere L, Nasr N, Arnaud C, et al. Prediction of delayed cerebral ischemia after subarachnoid hemorrhage using cerebral blood flow velocities and cerebral autoregulation assessment. *Neurocrit Care.* 2015;23(2):253–258.

18. Budohoski KP, Czosnyka M, Smielewski P, et al. Cerebral autoregulation after subarachnoid hemorrhage: comparison of three methods. *J Cereb Blood Flow Metab.* 2013;33(3):449–456.

19. Varsos GV, Budohoski KP, Czosnyka M, et al. Cerebral vasospasm affects arterial critical closing pressure. *J Cereb Blood Flow Metab.* 2014;35(2):285–291.

20. Dewey RC, Pieper HP, Hunt WE. Experimental cerebral hemodynamics. Vasomotor tone, critical closing pressure, and vascular bed resistance. *J Neurosurg.* 1974;41(5):597–606.

21. Varsos GV, Budohoski KP, Kolias AG, et al. Relationship of vascular wall tension and autoregulation following traumatic brain injury. *Neurocrit Care.* 2014;21(2):266–274.

22. Zweifel C, Czosnyka M, Carrera E, et al. Reliability of the blood flow velocity pulsatility index for assessment of intracranial and cerebral perfusion pressures in head-injured patients. *Neurosurgery.* 2012;71(4):853–861.

23. Swiat M, Weigele J, Hurst RW, et al. Middle cerebral artery vasospasm: transcranial color-coded duplex sonography versus conventional nonimaging transcranial Doppler sonography. *Crit Care Med.* 2009;37(3):963–968.

24. Vajkoczy P, Horn P, Thome C, et al. Regional cerebral blood flow monitoring in the diagnosis of delayed ischemia following aneurysmal subarachnoid hemorrhage. *J Neurosurg.* 2003;98(6):1227–1234.

25. Thome C, Vajkoczy P, Horn P, et al. Continuous monitoring of regional cerebral blood flow during temporary arterial occlusion in aneurysm surgery. *J Neurosurg.* 2001;95(3): 402–411.

26. Vajkoczy P, Roth H, Horn P, et al. Continuous monitoring of regional cerebral blood flow: experimental and clinical validation of a novel thermal diffusion microprobe. *J Neurosurg.* 2000;93(2):265–274.

27. Vajkoczy P, Horn P, Thome C, et al. Regional cerebral blood flow monitoring in the diagnosis of delayed ischemia following aneurysmal subarachnoid hemorrhage. *J Neurosurg.* 2003;98:1227–1234.

28. Hecht N, Fiss I, Wolf S, et al. Modified flow- and oxygen-related autoregulation indices for continuous monitoring of cerebral autoregulation. *J Neurosci Methods*. 2011;201(2): 399–403.

29. Barth M, Woitzik J, Weiss C, et al. Correlation of clinical outcome with pressure-, oxygen-, and flow-related indices of cerebrovascular reactivity in patients following aneurysmal SAH. *Neurocrit Care*. 2010;12(2):234–243.

30. Hoffman WE, Charbel FT, Edelman G, et al. Brain tissue oxygenation in patients with cerebral occlusive disease and arteriovenous malformations. *Br J Anaesth*. 1997;78(2): 169–171.

31. Charbel FT, Hoffman WE, Misra M, et al. Cerebral interstitial tissue oxygen tension, pH, HCO_3, CO_2. *Surg Neurol*. 1997;48(4):414–417.

32. Sarrafzadeh AS, Sakowitz OW, Callsen TA, et al. Bedside microdialysis for early detection of cerebral hypoxia in traumatic brain injury. *Neurosurg Focus*. 2000;9(5):e2.

33. Valadka AB, Gopinath SP, Contant CF, et al. Relationship of brain tissue PO_2 to outcome after severe head injury. *Crit Care Med*. 1998;26(9):1576–1581.

34. Rosenthal G, Hemphill JC, Sorani M, et al. Brain tissue oxygen tension is more indicative of oxygen diffusion than oxygen delivery and metabolism in patients with traumatic brain injury. *Crit Care Med*. 2008;36(6):1917–1924.

35. Menon DK, Coles JP, Gupta AK, et al. Diffusion limited oxygen delivery following head injury. *Crit Care Med*. 2004;32(6):1384–1390.

36. Claassen J, Perotte A, Albers D, et al. Nonconvulsive seizures after subarachnoid hemorrhage: multimodal detection and outcomes. *Ann Neurol*. 2013;74(1):53–64.

37. Jeon S-B, Choi HA, Badjatia N, et al. Hyperoxia may be related to delayed cerebral ischemia and poor outcome after subarachnoid haemorrhage. *J Neurol Neurosurg Psychiatry*. 2014;85(12):1301–1307.

38. Kilgannon JH, Jones AE, Shapiro NI, et al. Association between arterial hyperoxia following resuscitation from cardiac arrest and in-hospital mortality. *J Am Med Assoc*. 2010;303(21): 2165–2171.

39. Brenner M, Stein D, Hu P, et al. Association between early hyperoxia and worse outcomes after traumatic brain injury. *Arch Surg*. 2012;147(11):1042–1046.

40. Magnoni S, Ghisoni L, Locatelli M, et al. Lack of improvement in cerebral metabolism after hyperoxia in severe head injury: a microdialysis study. *J Neurosurg*. 2003;98:952–958.

41. Tolias CM, Reinert M, Seiler R, et al. Normobaric hyperoxia–induced improvement in cerebral metabolism and reduction in intracranial pressure in patients with severe head injury: a prospective historical cohort-matched study. *J Neurosurg*. 2004;101: 435–444.

42. Diringer MN. Hyperoxia—good or bad for the injured brain? *Curr Opin Crit Care*. 2008;14(2):167–171.

43. Diringer MN, Aiyagari V, Zazulia AR, et al. Effect of hyperoxia on cerebral metabolic rate for oxygen measured using positron emission tomography in patients with acute severe head injury. *J Neurosurg*. 2007;106(4):526–529.

44. Rockswold SB, Rockswold GL, Zaun DA, et al. A prospective, randomized phase II clinical trial to evaluate the effect of combined hyperbaric and normobaric hyperoxia on cerebral metabolism, intracranial pressure, oxygen toxicity, and clinical outcome in severe traumatic brain injury. *J Neurosurg*. June 2013;118(6):1317–1328.

45. Clifton GL, Valadka A, Zygun D, et al. Very early hypothermia induction in patients with severe brain injury (the National Acute Brain Injury Study: Hypothermia II): a randomised trial. *Lancet Neurol*. 2011;10(2):131–139.

46. Fletcher JJ, Bergman K, Blostein PA, et al. Fluid balance, complications, and brain tissue oxygen tension monitoring following severe traumatic brain injury. *Neurocrit Care.* 2010;13:47–56.

47. Budohoski KP, Czosnyka M, Smielewski P, et al. Impairment of cerebral autoregulation predicts delayed cerebral ischemia after subarachnoid hemorrhage: a prospective observational study. *Stroke.* 2012;43(12):3230–3237.

48. Marion DW, Puccio A, Wisniewski SR, et al. Effect of hyperventilation on extracellular concentrations of glutamate, lactate, pyruvate, and local cerebral blood flow in patients with severe traumatic brain injury. *Crit Care Med.* 2002;30(12):2619–2625.

49. Marcoux J, McArthur DA, Miller C, et al. Persistent metabolic crisis as measured by elevated cerebral microdialysis lactate-pyruvate ratio predicts chronic frontal lobe brain atrophy after traumatic brain injury. *Crit Care Med.* 2008;36(10):2871–2877.

50. Schmidt JM, Ko S-B, Helbok R, et al. Cerebral perfusion pressure thresholds for brain tissue hypoxia and metabolic crisis after poor-grade subarachnoid hemorrhage. *Stroke.* 2011;42(5):1351–1356.

51. Vespa P, McArthur DL, Stein N, et al. Tight glycemic control increases metabolic distress in traumatic brain injury: a randomized controlled within-subjects trial. *Crit Care Med.* 2012;40(6):1923–1929.

52. Vespa PM, Miller C, McArthur D, et al. Nonconvulsive electrographic seizures after traumatic brain injury result in a delayed, prolonged increase in intracranial pressure and metabolic crisis. *Crit Care Med.* 2007;35(12):2830–2836.

53. Gilmore EJ, Gaspard N, Choi HA, et al. Acute brain failure in severe sepsis: a prospective study in the medical intensive care unit utilizing continuous EEG monitoring. *Intensive Care Med.* 2015;41(4):686–694.

54. Claassen J, Jette N, Chum F, et al. Electrographic seizures and periodic discharges after intracerebral hemorrhage. *Neurology.* 2007;69(13):1356–1365.

55. Claassen J, Hirsch LJ, Frontera JA, et al. Prognostic significance of continuous EEG monitoring in patients with poor-grade subarachnoid hemorrhage. *Neurocrit Care.* 2006;4(2):103–112.

56. Claassen J, Hirsch LJ, Kreiter KT, et al. Quantitative continuous EEG for detecting delayed cerebral ischemia in patients with poor-grade subarachnoid hemorrhage. *Clin Neurophysiol.* 2004;115(12):2699–2710.

57. Kurtz P, Gaspard N, Wahl AS, et al. Continuous electroencephalography in a surgical intensive care unit. *Intensive Care Med.* 2014;40(2):228–234.

58. Oddo M, Carrera E, Claassen J, et al. Continuous electroencephalography in the medical intensive care unit. *Crit Care Med.* 2009;37(6):2051–2056.

59. Tao JX, Baldwin M, Hawes-Ebersole S, et al. Cortical substrates of scalp EEG epileptiform discharges. *J Clin Neurophysiol.* 2007;24(2):96–100.

60. Gaspard N, Hirsch LJ. Pitfalls in ictal EEG interpretation: critical care and intracranial recordings. *Neurology.* 2013;80(suppl 1):S26–S42.

61. Waziri A, Claassen J, Stuart RM, et al. Intracortical electroencephalography in acute brain injury. *Ann Neurol.* 2009;66(3):366–377.

62. Dreier JP, Woitzik J, Fabricius M, et al. Delayed ischaemic neurological deficits after subarachnoid haemorrhage are associated with clusters of spreading depolarizations. *Brain.* 2006;129(12):3224–3237.

63. Hartings JA, Bullock MR, Okonkwo DO, et al. Spreading depolarisations and outcome after traumatic brain injury: a prospective observational study. *Lancet Neurol.* 2011;10(12):1058–1064.

64. Dreier JP, Major S, Manning A, et al. Cortical spreading ischaemia is a novel process involved in ischaemic damage in patients with aneurysmal subarachnoid haemorrhage. *Brain*. 2009;132(pt 7):1866–1881.
65. Woitzik J, Dreier JP, Hecht N, et al. Delayed cerebral ischemia and spreading depolarization in absence of angiographic vasospasm after subarachnoid hemorrhage. *J Cereb Blood Flow Metab*. 2012;32(2):203–212.
66. Dreier JP, Major S, Pannek H-W, et al. Spreading convulsions, spreading depolarization and epileptogenesis in human cerebral cortex. *Brain*. 2012;135(pt 1):259–275.
67. Hertle DN, Dreier JP, Woitzik J, et al. Effect of analgesics and sedatives on the occurrence of spreading depolarizations accompanying acute brain injury. *Brain*. 2012;135(pt 8):2390–2398.
68. Drenckhahn C, Winkler MKL, Major S, et al. Correlates of spreading depolarization in human scalp electroencephalography. *Brain*. 2012;135(pt 3):853–868.
69. Chesnut R, Videtta W, Vespa P, et al. Intracranial pressure monitoring: fundamental considerations and rationale for monitoring. *Neurocrit Care*. 2014;21(suppl 2):S64–S84.

INDEX

"f" following page number indicates figure; "t" following page number indicates table.

CPSIA information can be obtained
at www.ICGtesting.com
Printed in the USA
LVOW06*0034200716
496933LV00003B/4/P

9 780813 579313